Being
On Top
of the World

Being
On Top
of the World

Toni Bobbin

Kangaroo Press

To my daughters, Louise and Amanda,
who have given me
love, joy, happiness and inspiration
and made my life worthwhile

First published in 1995 by Kangaroo Press Pty Ltd
3 Whitehall Road Kenthurst NSW 2156 Australia
PO Box 6125 Dural Delivery Centre NSW 2158
Printed in Hong Kong through Colorcraft Ltd

ISBN 0 86417 684 8

Contents

Introduction

This book has been written at Montville, a little craft village situated on the Blackall Range. I call it the TOP OF THE WORLD. Why? Because of the beauty of the emerald green fields, the picturesque homesteads, the quaint shops and restaurants. The spectacular Glasshouse Mountains lie to the south and in the eastern distance is the blue Pacific Ocean.

In winter pot-belly stoves burn sweet smelling pine cones, with thick steaming soups bubbling atop. In summer crisp delicious salads are served on rustic tables. The patios are overhung with creeping bougainvillea. It all belongs here. A winding ribbon of road runs from Mapleton to Maleny, with Montville taking pride of place between.

Here the soft green hills run down to the sea. Yes—this little bit of heaven is my Eden, my demi-Paradise.

—Toni Bobbin

Preface

Health is every individual's greatest responsibility. It is a divine gift which we should all enjoy for as long as we live. But health has many components which operate together to our benefit, and with which too many of us have lost touch.

I have written this book to help my readers adopt a healthy nutritious diet and healthy lifestyle. To choose an exercise programme. To alleviate stress—this chapter is important because people generally don't realise how badly stress can affect them.

Some people are born better looking than others, but we all have the potential to be more attractive than we are. The beauty chapter takes you one step at a time, teaching you to achieve a NEW YOU! Last but not least is happiness—one cannot be healthy if one is unhappy. The last chapter contains well over one hundred delicious recipes to help you take up your healthy nutritious diet.

Each day I would like you to make a plan and work out how you are going to spend your day, and how much time you are going to give each task, even if you can't realistically hope to accomplish them all in one day. Writing it down clears your mind of confusion. Include something you enjoy, like going to the beach, maybe a visit to the park, shopping, reading—whatever makes you feel good. It is too easy to get bogged down in life's daily demands and forget that at least one little daily indulgence is essential.

Learn something every day, even if it means looking a word up in the dictionary. When you go to bed, think, 'What did I learn today?' Do one thing you don't want to do, like writing that letter, phoning that person, sewing that hem; once it's done, you'll feel you have accomplished a great deal.

Keep your face and body looking good and your mind crystal clear. Look on the bright side of life and don't let stress get to you. Be positive, think, 'I look good, I feel great and, wet or fine, it's going to be a great day!'

Go ahead and enjoy...but before you start, take a moment to look at:

The Three Laws that Govern Life

All forms of animal life are governed by the three fundamental natural laws of nutrition, motion and oxidation. These laws are commonly referred to as eating, exercising and breathing.

Nutrition is the most important element of human life. Every time the clock ticks off a second the body has manufactured 2 500 000 new red blood cells. It produces nearly 150 million new blood cells every minute, and all the red blood cells in the body completely renew themselves every ninety days. Even as you read this page, yesterday's physical body has started to vanish. Your body of today is both appearing and disappearing. Tomorrow's blood, bones, glands and muscles are still to be created. The quality of next month's body is up to you, because your body chemistry is influenced by your food habits.

In terms of applied nutrition this means that through proper food selection one could be well on the way towards a healthier body and bloodstream within a very short time.

Nearly all the irregularities of the body are caused directly or indirectly by wrong eating. Correct eating is not alone the remedy for body irregularity but will render the body immune to most physical miseries. Of all the natural laws, nutrition is perhaps the least understood and most often violated.

CHAPTER 1 Dieting

Today I will try to live through this day only, not to tackle my whole life problem at once. I can do things for twelve hours that would appal me if I had to keep them up for a lifetime.

Today I will be happy. This assumes that what Abraham Lincoln said is true, that 'most folks are as happy as they make their minds up to be'. Happiness is from within; it is not a matter of externals.

Today I will try to adjust myself to what is, and not try to adjust everything to my own desires. I will take my family, my business and my life as they come and fit myself to them.

Today I will take care of my body. I will exercise it, care for it, nourish it, not abuse it nor neglect it, so that it will be perfect for my bidding.

Today I will strengthen my mind. I will learn something new and useful. I will not be a mental loafer. I will read something that requires effort, thought and concentration.

Today I will exercise my soul in three ways. I will do someone a good turn and not get found out. I will do at least two things I don't want to do, as William James suggests, just for exercise.

Today I will be agreeable. I will look as well as I can, dress as becomingly as possible, talk low, act courteously, be liberal with praise, criticise not at all, nor find fault with anything and not try to agitate nor improve anyone.

Today I will be unafraid, especially I will not be afraid to be happy, to enjoy what is beautiful, to love, and to believe that those I love, love me!

Anon.

Read on:

Diets and Slimming

For most of us slimming is a never-ending battle. We try to avoid dieting because—let's face it—rich food, salted and cooked in oil, smells and tastes so good. It's easy and fun to dine out and have takeaway, but one day you wake up and think, 'I AM FAT! NOW WHAT DO I DO?' You try to hide your body with bulky clothes; sure, this is okay for winter when you don't show much skin, but what about summer? You suddenly feel downhearted about yourself, frantically searching through your wardrobe to see what fits. You don't feel like going to the beach—no, there's no way you want to appear in your swimming costume. You feel

FAT AND UGLY!

You tackle the latest diet craze, do this for a couple of weeks and then begin to weaken. You dine out and have takeaway again, cheating here and there, having the odd cooked breakfast. Fried eggs, bacon, hash browns, served with thick buttered toast and jam, until finally you are back to your old ways and you plunge right back into the pangs of guilt and remorse. Until next time—then you start all over again.

CRASH DIETS JUST DON'T WORK!
THIS PROGRAMME DOES!

This is for life—not just for today or tomorrow, but always. You will lose weight, feel good and become a NEW YOU! Read the following pages carefully ...

How is your weight?

If you are overweight, you cannot be healthy and fit. Check your weight with the weight chart in this chapter. Remember bodies and builds vary, so make a small allowance for this.

You are overweight if:

- ❖ Your naked profile viewed in a mirror shows bulges in the wrong places.
- ❖ You can pinch 2.5 cm or more of loose flesh on upper arms, midriff or thighs.
- ❖ You can see fat shake when you jump up and down.

Let's begin

Weigh yourself once a week, midweek (every Wednesday); one tends to eat more on weekends. Weigh after getting up and going to the toilet, before showering or eating.

Use a graph to chart your loss: 1 kg a week is encouraging, but it can vary from one person to another. Buy a kilojoule counter to help you with your daily intake, or use a fat counter—fat grams are marked on all products. If you are doing any weight training or body sculpting, remember that muscle weighs more than fat. So don't be disheartened if your weight increases a little at first. You must keep to the kind of foods discussed on page 86 for your weight loss plan to work. Lie in bed at night and programme your subconscious mind, telling it you will be thin! You will be thin! WILL YOURSELF! Remember you can do anything you want to. Take a picture of your back view in bikini briefs. Put it on your mirror and in a few months' time take another one: hopefully you will see a big change, the NEW YOU!

How to reach your weight goal

If you are a woman aim to take in 6270 kilojoules* a day. If you are a man take in 9614 kilojoules a day. By the end of each week you should lose 1 kg. If you haven't, you are either not burning up sufficient kilojoules or you are cheating by eating the odd cake, meat pie, chips or whatever.

If you wish to lose weight faster

You will have to reduce your kilojoule intake:If you are a woman take in no more than 4180 kilojoules a day. If you are a man, no more than

*1 calorie = 4.18 kilojoules

7106 kilojoules a day. Keep to the programme and you could lose 4 kg per month. Make this your aim.

What you are aiming at!

Women			Men		
1.47 m 4'10"	47.5 kg	7 st 7 lb	1.57 m 5'2"	57 kg	9 st 0 lb
1.50 m 4'11"	48.5 kg	7 st 9 lb	1.60 m 5'3"	59 kg	9 st 4 lb
1.52 m 5'0"	50 kg	7 st 12 lb	1.63 m 5'4"	60.5 kg	9 st 7 lb
1.55 m 5'1"	51.5 kg	8 st 1 lb	1.65 m 5'5"	61.5 kg	9 st 10 lb
1.57 m 5'2"	52.5 kg	8 st 4 lb	1.68 m 5'6"	63 kg	9 st 13 lb
1.60 m 5'3"	54 kg	8 st 7 lb	1.70 m 5'7"	65 kg	10 st 3 lb
1.63 m 5'4"	56 kg	8 st 11 lb	1.73 m 5'8"	67 kg	10 st 8 lb
1.65 m 5'5"	57 kg	9 st 0 lb	1.75 m 5'9"	69 kg	10 st 12 lb
1.68 m 5'6"	59.5 kg	9 st 5 lb	1.78 m 5'10"	71 kg	11 st 2 lb
1.70 m 5'7"	61 kg	9 st 9 lb	1.80 m 5'11"	73 kg	11 st 7 lb
1.73 m 5'8"	63 kg	9 st 13 lb	1.83 m 6'0"	75 kg	11 st 11 lb
1.75 m 5'9"	65 kg	10 st 3 lb	1.85 m 6'1"	76.5 kg	12 st 1 lb
1.78 m 5'10"	66.5 kg	10 st 7 lb	1.88 m 6'2"	79 kg	12 st 6 lb
1.80 m 5'11"	68.5 kg	10 st 11 lb	1.90 m 6'3"	81 kg	12 st 11 lb
1.83 m 6'0"	70 kg	11 st 1 lb	1.93 m 6'4"	83.5 kg	13 st 2 lb

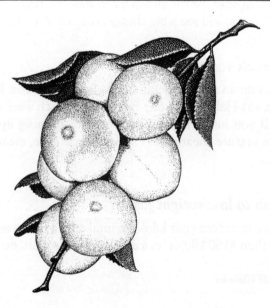

Activities Chart Showing Kilojoules Used per Minute

	kJ	cal.		kJ	cal.
Aerobics	33½	8	Horse riding	17	4
Archery	10½	2½	Ironing	under 2	under ½
Athletics	25	6	Jogging	21	5
Badminton	17	4	Judo	25	6
Basketball	25	6	Mountaineering	up to 42	up to 10
Bedmaking	10½	2½	Netball	21	5
Bends and			Polishing	10½	2½
stretches	10½	2½	Rollerskating	10½	2½
Bowls	10½	2½	Rowing	14½	3½
Canoeing	10½	2½	racing	up to 37½	up to 9
Cleaning	under 6	under 1½	Running	25	6
Climbing	17	4	Sailing	21	5½
Cricket—fielding,	under 6	under 1½	Scrubbing floors	23	5
batting, bowling	14½	3½	Shopping		
Croquet	10½	2½	(heavy load)	14½	3½
Cross-country			Skiing	23	5½
running	25	6	Skipping	33½	8
Cycling	17	4	Snooker	10½	2½
strenuous	33½	8	Squash	33½	8
Dancing	17	4	Swimming	33½	8
disco	25	6	Table tennis	10½	2½
Darts	under 6	under 1½	Tennis	14½	3½
Driving a car	under 6	1½	Trampolining	14½	3½
Dusting	6	1½	Vacuum cleaning	10½	2½
Fishing	6	1½	Volleyball	14½	3½
Gardening			Walking		
(heavy work)	21	5	comfortable pace	14½	3½
Golf	14½	3½	up stairs	17	4
Gymnastics	17	4	brisk walking	21	5
Hockey	17	4	Washing	under 6	under 1½
Home decorating	10½	2½	Water skiing	21	5

Example: If you jog for 10 minutes, you have used up 210 kilojoules.

Foods High in Kilojoules

Food	Measure	Kilojoules	Calories
Meat			
Steak— rump, average fat, grilled	100 g	1338	320
fillet, average fat, grilled	100 g	1588	380
T-bone, average fat, grilled	250 g	1880	450
Minced topside (one hamburger patty)	75 g	920	220
Lamb chop, short loin	60 g	940	225
Pork chop, grilled	70 g	1358	325
Bacon, one rasher	20 g	418	100
Dairy products			
Whole milk	30ml	84	20
Evaporated milk	1 tab	142	34
Flavoured milk	300 ml	920	220
Fruit yoghurt	200g ctn	794	190
Cheddar cheese	85 g	1505	360
Cheddar types grated	2 tabs	543	130
Cream cheese with added fruits	1 tabs	355	85
Cheese dips	1 tabs	250	60
Cream cheese	60 g	1045	250
Ice cream	1 scoop	376	90
Ice cream	1 litre	3762	900
Eggs, large	55 g	334	80
Butter/margarine	1 tsp	167	40
Polyunsaturated oils	1/2 cup	4180	1000
Sour cream	1½ tbs	397	95
Nuts			
Almonds, shelled	(26 nuts) 30 g	710	170
Beer nuts	30 g	710	170
Cashew nuts, roasted	(9 nuts) 30 g	752	180
Chestnuts	(5 nuts) 30 g	210	50
Macadamias	(9 nuts) 30 g	836	200
Mixed nuts	1 med pkt	2340	560

Food	Measure	Kilojoules	Calories
Biscuits and cakes			
Sweet biscuit	1	167	40
Chocolate biscuit	1	293	70
Apple slice	1	1045	250
Chocolate eclair	1	940	225
Chocolate cake	1 slice	940	225
Jam donut	1	1358	325
Croissant	1	1338	320
Scone	1	627	150
Bun	1	940	225
Lemon meringue pie	1 slice	1463	350
Chocolate mousse	1 serve	1672	400
Muesli slice	1	940	225
Chocolate bars			
Mars Bar	1	1380	330
Squares of chocolate	2 small	669	160
Block of chocolate	1 medium	1672	400
After-dinner mint	1	125	30
Box of chocolates	250 g	4598	1100
Jaffa	1	63	15
Caramel	1	104	25
Chewing-gum	1	42	10
Alcohol			
Wine, red or white	120 ml	334	80
Champagne	120 ml	397	95
Sherry	60 ml	376	90
Beer	10 oz (1 middy)	502	120
Shandy	10 oz	334	80
Spirits	60 ml (1 jigger)	585	140
Liqueurs	liqueur glass	250	60
Soft drinks			
Cola drinks	375 ml	656	157
Orange flavoured drinks	375 ml	836	200
Tonic water	375 ml	568	136
Flavoured mineral water	375 ml	627	150

Food	Measure	Kilojoules	Calories
Restaurant and takeaway foods			
Taco with meat, salad, cheese and			
sour cream	1	2508	600
Garlic prawns	1 serve	2090	500
Chinese lemon chicken	1 serve	2508	600
Chinese omelette (3 eggs and			
animal protein)	1 serve	3762	900
Fried rice	1 cup	1412	340
Sweet and sour fish	1 serve	5016	1200
Cannelloni with beef	1 serve	2299	550
Lasagne with beef	1 serve	2299	550
Spaghetti with beef	1 serve	2424	580
Lobster thermidor	1 serve	1881	450
Oysters in batter (fried)	6	961	230
Fried crumbed prawns	6	2236	535
Chips (French fries)	1 plateful	1965	470
Pork sausages	2	1385	325
Sausage roll	1	1463	350
Meat pie	1	2090	500
Pastie	1	1672	400
Fish and chips (battered and fried)	1 piece	1672	400
Chiko roll (fried)	1	1672	400
Potato scallop (fried)	1	1254	300

REMEMBER, 4180 KILOJOULES (1000 CALORIES) PER DAY

Eating Well in Ethnic Food

The recommended dishes, listed on pages 17–19, are generally lower in total fat, kilojoules and cholesterol than other dishes.

RIGHT: A beautiful view from the top of the Blackall Range at Montville, with the soft green hills running down to the sea and the mountains in the background

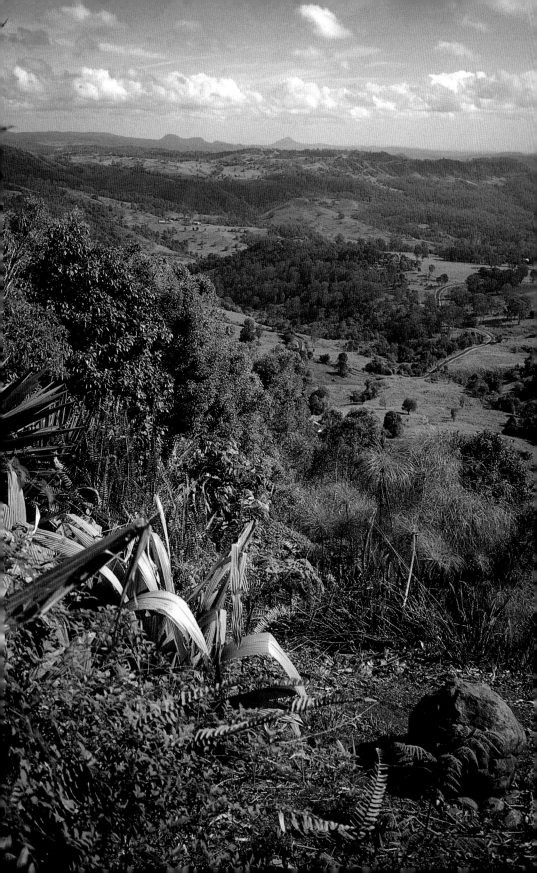

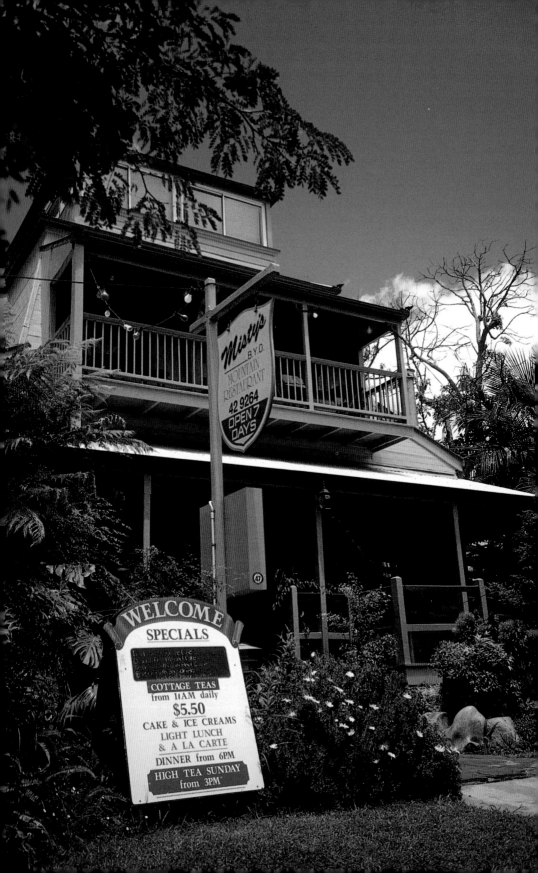

Recommended	Not recommended
Italian	
Pasta, vegetarian	Fettuccine alfredo
Cioppino (seafood soup)	Parmesan dishes
Steamed mussels in red sauce	Lasagne, cannelloni
Minestrone soup	Antipasto
Fruit ice	Garlic bread
Chinese	
White or brown rice	Fried rice
Moo goo gai pan	Crispy fried beef
Mixed vegetables (not fried)	Moo shu pork
Won ton soup	Fried won tons
Steamed dumplings	Sweet and sour pork
Mexican	
Steamed corn tortillas	Fried flour tortillas
Beans in soft tortilla	Beef enchiladas
Chicken with vegetables	Tortilla chips with guacamole
Black bean soup	Nachos
Gazpacho	Flautas
Japanese	
Sushi, sashimi	Tempura
Salmon steak	Tonkatsu (fried pork)
Miso soup	Torikatsu (fried chicken)
Chicken yakitori	Age tofu (fried tofu)
Indian	
Dal (lentils)	Puri (fried bread)
Vegetarian curries (go easy on the curries)	Coconut milk curry sauces
Pulka (unleavened bread)	Samosa (fried appetisers)
Basmati rice with vegetables	Muglai (creamy curry sauce)

Beware of hidden fats and calories in many ethnic dishes.

LEFT: *Misty's Restaurant, Montville*

Chinese

When dining Chinese choose seafood or a steamed vegetable dish; allow yourself small portions served with generous helpings of plain boiled rice. (One order is often enough for two: don't *over order*). Snow peas with water chestnuts and bamboo shoots are a good bet (1484 kJ with rice). Stay away from such dishes as crispy beef (1948 kJ with rice).

Italian

Skip the antipasto and garlic bread, stick with the Italian bread. Have a green salad with a low oil and vinegar dressing (1 part oil, 3 parts vinegar). Steamed mussels are a good choice. Watch out for olive oil (502 kJ a tablespoon). Cheese is laden with kilojoules and fat; opt for a tablespoon of parmesan (96 kJ); sprinkled over a low-fat pasta dish. Calamari stewed with vegetables is a good low calorie dish (878 kJ); cannelloni is one of the worst (3402 kJ).

Mexican

Keep it simple. A plain tostada has only 250 kJ, but add meat, beans, sour cream, avocado and cheese and your 250 kJ become 1379 kJ. Stay with beans, lettuce, tomato and salsa as toppings, and you limit the fat and kilojoules. Soups are usually a good choice, but forgo the sour cream on top. Avoid the fried foods. Chicken tacos are a good choice, only 957 kJ each. Enchiladas (meat, cheese and sour cream) are one of the worst choices with 1919 kJ each. Request corn tortillas instead of flour tortillas.

Indian

Because vegetarian dishes are abundant in Indian cuisine, finding low-fat food is relatively easy but you should still proceed with caution. The amount of oil used, even in vegetarian curries, varies greatly. Steer clear of fried appetisers like samosas and paboris and fried bread like puri. Rather try the mulligatawny soup (made from lentils), baked bread (nan) and the sweet and sour cabbage. Yoghurt-based dishes may be a good option if the yoghurt is low in fat. Choose vegetable curries over meat ones. Dal palak, a split pea dish, provides 957 kJ a serve, including rice, whereas a creamy beef curry made with coconut milk is 2153 kJ a serve.

Japanese

Japanese food is usually low in fat, but high in sodium. Pickled vegetables (ishinko) served as appetisers are fat-free but high in salt. Clear soups are a good choice. Yakitori steamed chicken pieces served on a skewer provide 1149 kJ. By comparison a small serving of tonkatsu, a fried pork chop, provides a singular 1124 kJ a serving, but half the kilojoules come from fat. A safe choice is shabu-shabu, a tray of meat or seafood and vegetables cooked by dipping in boiling broth. Tofu-based dishes are also a good bet, with the exception of fried tofu.

An Example of What Not to Eat

A 'Special Sunday Treat' can amount to 25 073 kilojoules in one day!

	Kilojoules	Calories
Breakfast		
1 glass sweetened apple juice	313	75
2 large fried eggs	669	160
3 bacon rashers	1254	300
1 grilled tomato	460	110
1 serve hash brown potatoes	1129	270
2 slices white toast with butter	961	230
2 cups coffee with milk and sugar	376	90
	5162	**1235**
Morning tea		
1 finger bun with butter	1965	470
1 cup coffee with milk and sugar	188	45
	2153	**515**
Lunch		
1 hamburger with the lot	2299	550
1 large chips	1374	330
1 apple pie	1086	260
1 chocolate milkshake	1149	275
	5908	**1415**

	Kilojoules	Calories
Afternoon tea		
2 sweet cream biscuits	376	90
2 cups coffee with milk and sugar	418	100
	794	**190**
Cocktail hour		
4 middies of beer	2006	480
1 packet of beer nuts	2090	500
	4096	**980**
Dinner		
2 glasses of wine	669	160
1 T-bone steak	1881	450
1 baked potato with sour cream	690	165
Greek salad with dressing	899	215
1 piece pavlova and cream	2090	500
1 Irish coffee	731	175
	6960	**1665**
Total for day	**25073**	**6 000**

A dramatic demonstration of how to eat and become overweight!

An Example of What to Eat

This weight-loss daily diet suggestion amounts to 4180 kilojoules for one day.

	Kilojoules	Calories
Breakfast		
Fruit salad	272	65
1 chopped apple	334	80
1 sliced banana	167	40
1 kiwi fruit	42	10
Herb tea	0	0
	815	**195**

	Kilojoules	Calories
Morning tea		
Herb tea	0	0
2 slices pineapple	251	60
	251	**60**
Lunch		
Pita bread	313	75
Filling		
½ avocado	284	68
grated carrot	134	32
sliced tomato	84	20
chopped lettuce	8	2
chopped onion	63	15
alfalfa sprouts	42	10
Herb tea	0	0
	928	**222**
Afternoon tea		
1 carton low fat yoghurt	460	110
1 banana	334	80
	794	**190**
Dinner		
Pumpkin soup	209	50
Poached chicken breast in white wine	522	125
Fresh steamed asparagus	251	60
Wild rice	201	48
½ grilled tomato	209	50
Herb tea	0	0
	1392	**333**
Total for day	**4180**	**1000**

The Ten Dont's of Dieting

1. **DON'T** get hungry. Eat some vegetable sticks, salad or chopped fruit. Have these things ready prepared; there is no excuse for bad planning. In the morning or evening chop up some zucchini, carrots, celery, capsicum sticks and keep them in an airtight container in the refrigerator. When you go to the fridge for the usual cheese and cold cuts snacks, eat the sticks instead.
2. **DON'T** eat breakfast cereals, including muesli and porridge. They are acid forming and hard to digest—eat fruit instead; remember, it digests in two hours.
3. **DON'T** crash diet, it's unwise. Single-item diets featuring bananas, water or grapefruit, for example, or high protein diets, promising the loss of 3.5 kg in a week are dangerous; most of the weight loss results from losing extra water. In fact you haven't lost any fat at all, you are merely dehydrated!
4. **DON'T** eat chocolate bars, cakes and biscuits. If you cheat, go for a brisk half hour's walk, jog or rebound for twenty minutes.
5. **DON'T** give in. Remember you will lose more weight in the first week than you will in the following ones because you will lose extra liquid from your body in the first week as well as breaking down fat.
6. **DON'T** mix drinking and dieting. Alcohol lowers your inhibitions and muddles your judgment and is also high in kilojoules. If you must have the odd social drink, mix it half and half; for example, half a glass of wine mixed with half a glass of soda water or mineral water, with lots of ice.
7. **DON'T** drink coffee or any caffeinated beverages. These affect your blood sugar. Coffee even when decaffeinated contains a substance which makes you feel hungry.
8. **DON'T** think constantly of cooked food. Instead of a large plate of beef casserole try a delicious plate of crisp salad vegetables; get away from the cooking pot.
9. **DON'T** eat a lot of dried fruit and nuts. Both are very high in kilojoules; for example, dried raisins are 600% higher in kilojoules than an equal weight of fresh grapes.
10. **DON'T** binge. When you are feeling lonely and downhearted, eat your prepared vegetable sticks, salad or chopped fruit pieces and programme yourself to be happy!

The Importance of Water

1. Buy yourself a water purifier (tap water is loaded with chemicals)
2. Water satisfies hunger pangs
3. Water helps reduce cellulite
4. Water helps flush waste products (toxins) and fat from your system

Drink 8-12 glasses (2 litres) of water daily. If water haters find this hard going at first, here is a tip: fill a jug with 2 litres of water, squeeze in some freshly juiced lemon and add ice cubes; keep it in the fridge and drink throughout the day. Herbal teas can be counted as part of your daily intake. Hot water is surprisingly palatable on a cold day.

People who eat a lot of fruit and vegetables (high water-content foods) each day are washing toxic wastes from their body, thus decreasing their weight plus getting the benefit of detoxifying their bodies.

People who eat large amounts of concentrated foods (for example, meats and cereals), will need to drink a lot more than 2 litres of water at first. But after a few weeks your daily water consumption will be lowered. Remember, always drink distilled water as tap water is loaded with chemicals.

Don't drink water with your meals; this dilutes the stomach juices and stops the food from being properly digested.

Peace at Meal Time

Organise your meal times so you eat in peace. Think of a deer grazing; the moment it senses danger it stops eating. This reaction to disturbance is a natural process. You know yourself that if you have an argument at the dining table it becomes hard to swallow your food. The reason is that the brain sends a biological message which instantly turns you off your food.

Avoid TV trays on laps and turn the television off. Set the table with a clean cloth, napkins and fresh flowers, maybe dim the lights, turn on some soothing music. Relax and enjoy your meal in peace and, don't forget, serve yourself a small helping! Eat slowly and chew your food well. All these things help you appreciate your food more and help your body utilise it better.

CHAPTER 2

Exercise

> By chase our fathers earned their food;
> Toil strung their hearts and purified their blood,
> But we their sons, a pampered race of men,
> Are dwindled down to three score years and ten,
> Better to hunt in fields, for health unbought,
> Than fee the doctor for a nauseous draught.
> The wise, for cure, on exercise depend;
> God never made His work for man to mend.

John Dryden, 1680

To introduce my exercise chapter I wish to quote a paragraph from Mildred Cooper's book titled *Aerobics for Women*. She writes:

> *One night Ken and I were relaxing after dinner watching television and he said, 'Take my resting heart rate?' So I checked his pulse and got 50 beats a minute. Then he counted mine and got 80 beats. 'Thirty beats difference isn't much,' I said blithely. 'Oh no? Think of it this way,' said my cagey husband. 'While we're asleep tonight, your heart is going to beat about ten thousand times more than mine will. Even though our hearts are pumping the same amount of blood, it takes your heartbeat that much more work and effort to do the job because you're not in condition. You're just going to wear out faster than I will.' Do I need to elaborate on what went through my head, including visions of Ken, a widower, courting the woman who would become the second Mrs Cooper and Berkley's stepmother?*

> *The combination of these dire thoughts with the fact that deep down inside, I secretly admitted Ken was right about the need for daily exercise and the benefits of it, finally persuaded me that I couldn't afford not to get into an aerobics conditioning programme...*

I think this should inspire anyone to feel enthusiastic about beginning an aerobics programme.

Any exercise is better than none, and frequent light exercise is of more benefit than bursts of vigorous exercise with extended periods of inactivity between them.

The main benefit of exercise is gained from movement, because it is muscular movement that boosts the circulation of the body fluids which take nourishment to the tissue cells and at the same time cleanse them by removing their waste products for elimination.

The extra benefit of regular sustained vigorous (aerobic) exercise is that it not only enhances the entire circulation of the body's blood and lymph fluids, but allows excess blood fats, derived from too much fat in the diet, to be used up as fuel for the muscles. With the removal of this fat the blood becomes more fluid and circulates more freely, lowering the heart's workload and lowering the blood pressure.

Athletes in regular training can thus escape to a great extent the onset of many common diseases, the most dangerous of which are heart disease and cancer.

The benefits of exercise can be achieved by quite moderate activity. It should never be continued to a state bordering on distress or exhaustion, in which case the extra effort is wasted and is sometimes dangerous.

Please don't let flagging spirits and a lack of energy be an excuse for chomping on a chocolate bar. Research has proven that a brisk twelve-minute walk or jog provides more sustained energy than consuming a bar of chocolate and, what's more, it reduces tension, aids toning and increases weight loss. This book's weight loss programme will not work without exercise—no weight loss programme will.

❖ Exercise eases pain and helps you beat the blues. Research shows increasing respect for physical activity. The hormones that exercise releases lift the spirits and erase many aches and pains. Exercise also calms your nerves in stressful situations—for example, when you are under pressure caused by such things as taking an exam or being constantly nagged, go for a jog or brisk walk and let your body calm itself down.
❖ Exercise helps with slimming and confidence building; it helps you deal with major problems, including surplus weight. When you exercise you are less inclined to binge—being busy you'll forget about food!

❖ Exercise is a must for post-menopausal women. Women during childbearing years have the advantage of the female hormone oestrogen which offers a level of protection against heart disease. They have traditionally ranked behind men in deaths from heart disease, because of this hormone. When women enter the menopause the level of oestrogen declines, leaving them open to heart disease. Aerobic exercise helps keep your heart in top condition.

❖ Exercise helps you to sleep soundly; your body is more relaxed after exercise and tension is reduced.

❖ Exercise does much to minimise the risks of heart disease, but very few Australians are active at work or during leisure hours. We as a nation have one of the highest rates of heart disease in the world and are amongst the fattest people in the world.

THE BEST FORM OF EXERCISE IS AN AEROBIC ONE!

The word *aerobic* refers to a process such as respiration which is dependent on molecular oxygen or air. An aerobic exercise is any activity that promotes the delivery of oxygen to the cells, such as jogging, cycling, swimming, skipping, brisk walking, rebounding, aerobics classes.

The word *anaerobic* refers to a process where energy is obtained without oxygen. Anaerobic activities include golf, squash, slow walking, gardening, or any exercise in which you stop and start. These exercises are not heartbuilding.

Aerobic exercise is the best form of exercise to adopt to keep yourself in tip-top condition and strengthen your heart.

Ideas for Your Aerobic Exercise Programme

Skipping

Skip for 15 minutes each day. This will help to reduce high blood pressure. Try to get into a daily routine, just like brushing your teeth each morning.

Rebounding

This is my favourite and a great way of exercising. You can buy a mini trampoline at any variety store, such as KMart, for about fifty dollars. Store it under a bed, or in a spare room, when not in use. Why not rebound to music? Take it out into the garden, enjoy the sunshine and fresh air and rebound. Start with five minutes and build up your time by five minute intervals until you can manage twenty minutes. All ages can enjoy it. Rebounding tones and strengthens the cells in your body as it works against the gravitational pull. If you wish to learn more about rebounding purchase a copy of *The Miracles of Re-bound Exercise* by Albert E. Carter.

Brisk walking

Did you know you burn as many calories walking briskly for one mile as you do running it? Plus you get to enjoy the scenery, sunshine and flowers. If you are visiting another city you can walk and appreciate the buildings, atmosphere and feel of the place. You must walk fast enough and long enough, fifteen minutes would be the minimum, to get your *heart working aerobically*. Park your car some distance from your destination and walk the rest of the way; if you are travelling by public transport you could do the same thing. Brisk walk for twenty minutes—ten minutes from home, ten minutes back.

Jogging

Jog a mile along the beach. Make sure the tide is low as the sand must be hard; soft sand can damage ankles and knees. If you work, jog around the park in your lunch break; try to avoid busy streets teeming with traffic and exhaust fumes. Beat the pollution.

Aerobics

Nearly all suburbs and country towns have a gym where aerobics classes are held. Book into the class and attend three times a week (more if possible); you will meet new friends who will inspire you to keep attending while you are becoming fit and trimming down your body.

Roving

The Pritikin Programme calls this exercise 'roving': you walk or run according to how you feel, starting with a couple of blocks, and with improving condition extend to 10–15 km (6–10 miles), three days a week or whatever. Distance is important, time is not.

WARNINGS

People with a heart condition or high blood pressure **must** consult their doctor before embarking on any exercise programme.

Under 30: You can start immediately, providing you are medically fit.

30-49: Seek a medical if you intend to do vigorous exercises.

50-59: Condition yourself with a walking programme before you contemplate anything more strenuous. Have a medical checkup before jogging, cycling, etc.

Over 60: Walking, stationary cycling, rebounding and swimming are encouraged.

Do not exercise if you have a bad cold or sore throat, flu symptoms or a temperature.

Questions before starting:

1. Have you recently had a baby?
2. Do you suffer from chest pains associated with effort?
3. Do you have heart trouble or high blood pressure?
4. Do you ever have dizzy spells or feel faint?
5. Do you have a back problem?
6. Are you a heavy smoker?
7. Have you recently had a serious illness or operation?

If any of the answers are yes, consult your doctor before beginning your exercise programme.

The Point System

Kenneth Cooper in his book *Aerobics* has a point system; to get regular exercise you must 'earn' 30 points per week. He gives point values to various forms of exercise:

> 1 mile (1.6 km) walked or run in under $14^1/_2$ minutes gets 2 points
> 1 mile (1.6 km) walked or run in under 12 minutes gets 3 points
> 1 mile (1.6 km) walked or run in under 10 minutes gets 4 points
> Swimming 500 yards (450 metres) in $12^1/_2$ minutes gets 4 points.

You could graph out your own point system to equal 30 points per week.

Remember exercise is the name of the game! You will look and feel younger, your waist will be thinner, your hips and thighs firmer, and best of all you will be permanently rid of many kilograms of fat. Inactivity can kill you!!

Let's Begin

1. Exercise in the cool if possible. Drink plenty of water.
2. Do not exercise within two hours of eating—exercise before meals instead.
3. Build up your exercise programme slowly.
4. If you are on blood pressure medication or medication to slow down your heart DO NOT attempt any exercise programme without your doctor's approval.
5. Warm down at the end of an exercise.
6. Try to exercise in the early morning; the air is crisper and your body fitter then.
7. One way to measure fitness is to check your pulse rate. Place the tips of your first two fingers (not your thumb) at the side of your throat or on your wrist. Count the beats for 30 seconds, then multiply by two to get the total per minute—your pulse rate. Take your resting pulse rate first thing in the morning, before getting out of bed.

What the readings mean:

over 90	=	unfit
80–90	=	below average
70–80	=	average
60–70	=	fit
under 60	=	very fit

Note: Pulse rates for smokers will be 5 to 10 beats higher.

8. As a further indicator of your fitness level, get up slowly, stand for about 30 seconds and take your pulse rate again. Note the difference between this and the previous rate.
   A difference of:

over 15 beats	=	unfit
12–14 beats	=	below average
8–11 beats	=	average
4–7 beats	=	fit
1–3 beats	=	very fit

Step test

Use the bottom step of a staircase. Step up with your left foot, then your right, then down with your left foot, then your right. Do a test run to get the footwork right and to check your pace, then step up 24 times a minute for 3 minutes. Stop; wait 1 minute, take your pulse. These are the ratings for women:

under 76 beats per minute	=	excellent
76–85 beats per minute	=	good
86–94 beats per minute	=	average
95–110 beats per minute	=	below average

Note: You are not fit if you cannot run for a bus without being winded; can't walk briskly with people your own age, matching their pace and carrying on a conversation; can't climb 20 stairs without stopping to get your breath.

Once you have decided on what exercise is best for you, try to stick to a certain time each day.

Here are some different ways to help you make a move: Jog along the beach or street; plan a little run around your yard—ten times or so. Rebound for twenty minutes? Walk for thirty minutes. You may wish to skip, cycle or swim each day. After you become fit remember your heart will have a lot less work to do. What is twenty minutes taken out of a twenty-four hour day? (You could spend this time chatting on the phone.) Why not rebound while you're having that chat?

At the end of your exercise:
1. Sit down and rest for one minute; don't overdo it.
2. Take your pulse rate. Count for 60 seconds (or 30 seconds and double it).
3. If your pulse is more than 130 beats per minute the exercise was too strenuous. A count of 100 beats per minute indicates a good level of fitness.

The rewards of exercise:
❖ Weight control
❖ Reduced stress
❖ Muscle tone
❖ Appetite control
❖ Lower blood pressure
❖ Increased heart and lung efficiency
❖ Less sleepless nights

All gained from 20 minutes exercise three or four days a week. GO FOR IT!

Daily Exercises for Problem Areas

These exercises won't make you lose weight but they will help remove the flab and make muscles stronger and firmer. They are as simple as A, B, C. ('Only five minutes a day to trim the fat away!')
A: Three exercises for the waist.
B: Three exercises for the stomach.
C: Three exercises for the bottom.

Warm up first!
1. Reach up as high as you can with one arm with your hand directly

31

over your head. When you feel all stretched out drop your arm. Repeat the exercise with other arm. *(10 times)*

2. Lie flat on the floor and do ten pushups; or touch toes ten times.

The stretching will get your blood circulating. When doing the exercises, breathe deeply, hold your breath for five seconds and exhale.

A: *The Waist*

EXERCISE 1
Stand with feet apart, both hands clenched on waist, elbows bent, twist your body in either direction as far as you can turn—left, right, left, right and so on. *(10 times)*

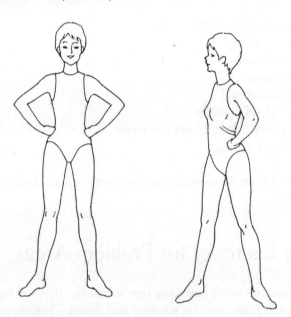

EXERCISE 2
Sit in the lotus position (or half lotus), back erect, fingers clasped behind head. Thrust upper body from waist to right. Lower left elbow to right knee. Untwist and lift to starting position. Repeat to left. *(5 each side)*

RIGHT: *Warm up with a few stretches before you begin your exercise session*

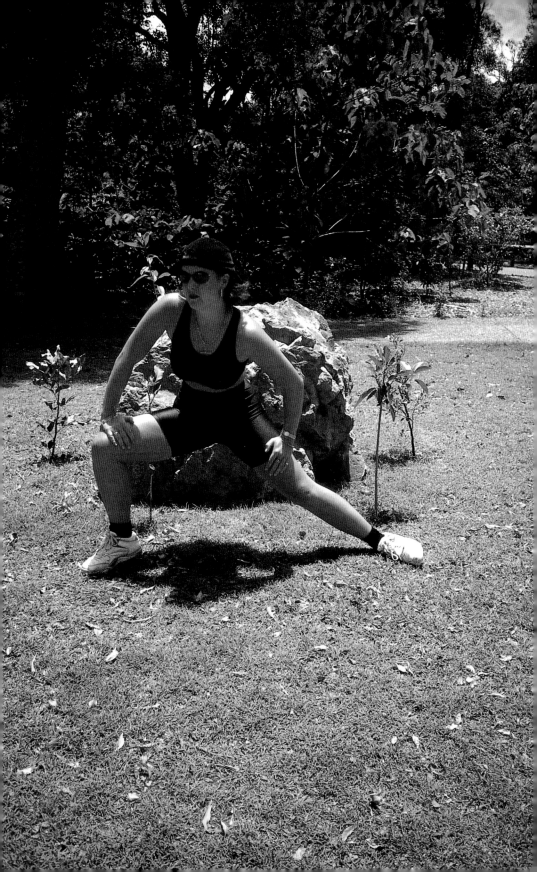

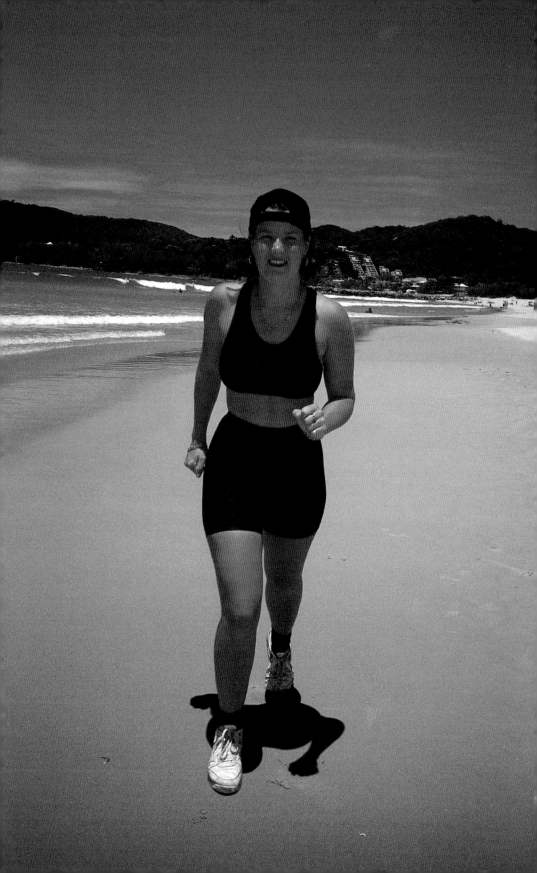

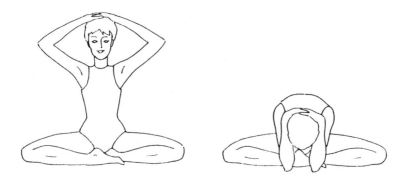

Lower head and bring elbows together. Hold for 8. Uncurl. Repeat sequence. *(4 times)*

EXERCISE 3
Sit with left knee bent and resting on floor. Rest left heel against right buttock, arms relaxed. Cross right foot over left thigh. Twist upper body from waist to your left, place right hand on right heel and left palm behind on floor. Hold for count of 20. *(Repeat twice each side)*

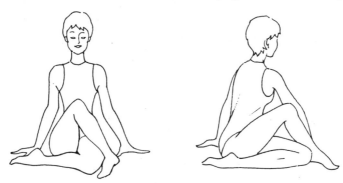

B: The Stomach

EXERCISE 1
Lie flat on the floor. Lift legs apart about 30 cm above the floor, pedal as if you were pedalling a bicycle, repeat. *(20 times)*

LEFT: *Jogging along the uncrowded Noosa Heads beach*

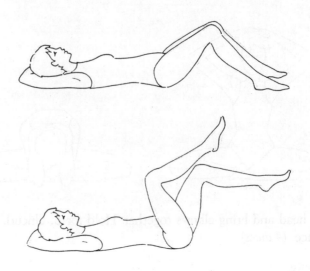

EXERCISE 2

Begin on hands and knees (all fours); place hands shoulder width apart, back straight. Round your back, lower your head, and contract your stomach muscles. Hold for the count of 5. Return to start, repeat. *(10 times)*

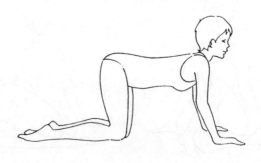

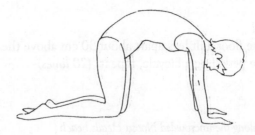

EXERCISE 3

Lie on floor, arms outstretched behind head and knees bent, raise arms, lean towards ankles and clasp them. Relax back, repeat. *(10 times)*

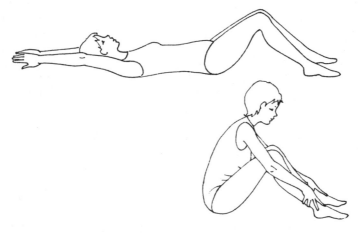

Other methods for stomach and cellulite

1. If you have the time to spare, and the money, invest in a G5 treatment from your beautician to break down cellulite. You would need three sessions, with twelve treatments each session. The total cost would be about $300.

2. Each morning under the shower rub your stomach and thighs with a stiff brush or loofah. You can also roll them with a small roller made especially for the job. Drink plenty of water to get rid of the waste products from your body.

C: *The Bottom*

EXERCISE 1

Stand with your left hand on the back of a chair or table for support. Bring your right leg out to the side, foot raised so only your toes touch the floor, move your foot along the floor until it is behind your left leg. Still keeping your toes on the floor, return your leg to the starting position. *(10 times each leg)*

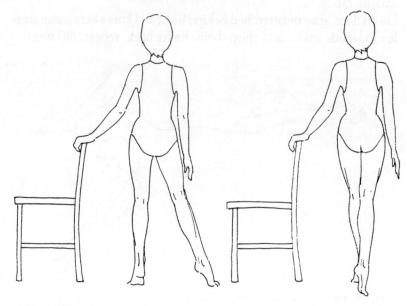

EXERCISE 2
Clench and unclench buttocks ten times (do it hard!) at any spare
moment when you are standing around. You'll help fight the sag and
flabbiness.

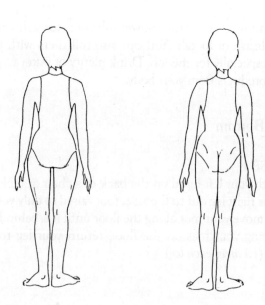

EXERCISE 3

Hold onto the back of a chair. Stand with your legs apart and feet flat, start to sit down, keeping your feet flat on the ground. Stop the moment just before your bottom reaches the ground. Hold the position for a few seconds and then gradually bring your knees and feet together. *(10 times)*

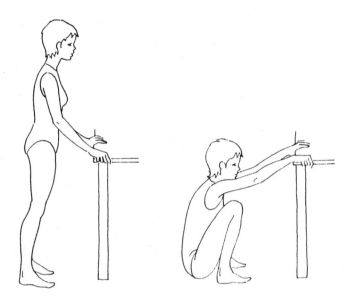

You'll be doing a total of nine exercises. It shouldn't take more than five or ten minutes each morning. As you become more flexible, increase the number of repeats.

CHAPTER 3 Stress

How blessed is he, who leads a country life,
Unvex'd with anxious cares, and void of strife!
Who studying peace, and shunning civil rage,
Enjoy'd his youth, and now enjoys his age.

John Dryden

Stress is the effect upon a subject when a situation requires them to adapt to it or to take avoiding action. The influence can be emotional or physical but not necessarily harmful or threatening. Whatever the cause, stress evokes physiological responses in the body. Factors which cause stress are called stressors.

Dr Hans Selye, author of The Stress of Life *and* Stress Without Distress *and perhaps the most experienced researcher on the subject, says factors such as fear, sorrow, joy, excitement, heat, cold or drugs, elicit in the body identical bio-chemical reactions. Whether the influence is pleasant or unpleasant is immaterial; the reaction depends only upon the intensity of the demand to adapt and the duration of the demand. However, the stress caused by elation, which Dr Selye calls eustress (eu = good), causes less damaging effects because the body readily adapts.*

In his evolutionary past, man has always had to contend with a certain amount of stress of one kind or another and his body evolved to react properly to it as a normal event. Just as man's body over eons of primitive environment developed to function on simple natural food, so it developed to cope with the stresses of a simple natural lifestyle. These no doubt would often have been quite severe but usually of brief duration and never in great profusion. Not only can the body easily contend with a moderate or normal amount of stress, it actually thrives upon its stimulating effect.

When levels of stress reach a point where the body can no longer cope easily, the effect becomes harmful and as Dr Selye says, the condition becomes one of distress. Thus to refer to stress as being harmful is misleading, it is the condition of distress which is harmful.

Ross Horne, The Health Revolution

Stressful Events

If any of these events have occurred in your life recently, add the points for each event. If your score within the last year is 150, there would be a good 50% chance of becoming ill within the next two years. With a total of 300 the probability is 80%.

	Points out of 100
Death of spouse	100
Divorce	73
Marital separation	65
Jail term	63
Death of a close family member	63
Personal injury or illness	53
Marriage	50
Fired from work	47
Marital reconciliation	45
Retirement	45
Change in family member's health	44
Pregnancy	40
Sex difficulties	39
Addition to family	39
Business readjustment	39
Change in financial status	38
Death of a close friend	37
Change to different line of work	36
Mortgage loan	31
Foreclosure of mortgage loan	30
Son or daughter leaving home	29
Trouble with illness	29
Outstanding personal achievement	28
Spouse begins or stops work	26
Starting or finishing school	25
Trouble with boss	23
Change in work hour conditions	20
Change in residence	20
Change in schools	20
Change in church activities	19
Change in sleeping habits	16
Change in number of family gatherings	15

Change in eating habits	15
A holiday	13
Christmas season	12
Minor violation of law	11

Figures taken from Dr Holmes, *Rahe Survey* (University of Washington Medical School)

Avoiding Stress and Feeling Happy

The Rules

1. Live for today and forget the past. The way to achievement lies in letting go and reaching out for the future. If you can't look forward to each day you must look back and to look back, as Lot's wife found out, is to become a pillar of salt, not much use to anybody. One can't change what has happened. Don't let resentments and regrets ruin the present. Live each day as it comes and enjoy it to the fullest. Take the risks; the person who risks nothing does nothing, is nothing.

2. Don't put off decisions. If you have a problem or a decision to make tackle it. First look thoroughly into the problem, write down the steps you should take and go ahead and take them. List the things you can do, when and how you can do them, then move; be positive and determined.

3. It is hard to change other people. If you have an argument with a family member, friend or boss, keep calm, don't scream; count to ten, smile inwardly, then later congratulate yourself on doing a good job. Don't let people get to you; say you are driving along and some person shouts abuse because of your careless driving, then wave, blow them a kiss—it works wonders!

4. Ask yourself, just what am I worried about? Is it my job or no job, my marriage, my children, my parents, my money, my weight, my drug habits, a friend, illness, loneliness? Be exact, pinpoint the problem. Write down actual details. If it's money ask yourself, what am I doing with my money? Am I wasting it? Now what am I going to do about it? Solution: Create a budget and keep to it. If you can't work out your own problems, seek advice from a professional such as a counsellor, lawyer, clergyman, hypnotist or

naturopath to reorganise you life. Always remember, all the worry in the world won't make the slightest difference. Call it what you wish—fate or karma—90% of what we worry about *doesn't happen anyway*. Worry is wasted energy.

5. Often worry exists only in your imagination. It is so easy to imagine a whole world of fears, excitements, failures, all without moving from your living room. When you feel overwhelmed by pointless worry for yourself and others, look at it closely; remind yourself of the difference between reality and fantasy. Replace the worry with constructive, pleasant thoughts and actions.

6. When you become older, don't give up. You can act and feel sixteen at sixty (and then again you can act sixty at sixteen). Don't think, 'I am a senior citizen.' Think, 'I am a woman.' 'I am a man.' Enjoy your life to the utmost. How old would you be if you didn't know how old you were!

7. Think seriously about your shortcomings; don't put the blame on your dear parents, your spouse, your friends, teachers, bosses or society. *It is up to you!* Maybe you have had some rough patches but that's part of the learning process. Try to learn from your mistakes, for out of something bad comes something good. 'As ye sow, so shall ye reap.'

8. Learn to look at life with a huge beaming smile on your face, laugh and that sense of humour will come smiling through. 'Laughter is the best kind of medicine.'

9. Say to yourself, 'I don't like it! But I can handle it!'

10. And remember for the rest of your life, 'There is always someone less fortunate than yourself.'

Stress can upset the hormonal balance of the body. The blood flow becomes sluggish and the blood becomes thick, thus making circulation difficult. This can lead to physical illnesses such as head colds, flu, skin rashes, ulcers, heart disease and cancer. The warning signs are there, telling you to SLOW DOWN! Take a good look at yourself, your diet, exercise programme, recreation, drug habits and medical pills.

Have strength of mind.

DON'T let it be too late!
DON'T say, 'Why me?'

41

If your stress level is high, along with your fatty food intake, you have bad drug habits and nothing is being done to rectify the problem, you could be dead sooner than you think! Maybe the stress has passed but your drug habits have remained? Of course your best friends won't tell you! The sooner you adopt a healthy programme the better.

Once the stress is removed, the cholesterol in the blood is reduced, the oxygen to the cells improves and the hormonal balance is restored, you'll feel like a new person and live a lot longer.

Nobody Wants Distress!

It's the lucky person who can go through life without an unhappy experience.

Some people cope well with difficult situations, others throw up their hands in desperation, not knowing which way to turn. Let's take Johnny, for example, who has become dependent on various forms of drugs. He is worried about the repayments on his house and whether his car will be repossessed or not.

Johnny wakes feeling depressed; he misses breakfast and takes one of his happy pills (anti-depressant tablets) followed by a couple of headache pills to help fight the hangover from the night before, drinks a glass of water, Alka-Seltzer in it, slumps down to a cup of tea/coffee and a cigarette. During the morning he smokes more cigarettes and drinks several more cups of tea/coffee. Operating on about 50% brain power, he is clumsy at work. Lunch usually consists of a couple of meat pies or hamburgers followed by a cream bun and a bottle of soft drink loaded with sugar and caffeine.

After work he heads for the pub and has quite a few beers along with more cigarettes and another happy pill. If he makes it home for dinner he eats steak or sausages, chips and a veg. He settles down to watch TV, sipping along on a few more beers. Before going to bed he takes a sleeping tablet and finally falls into a drugged sleep.

Next morning Johnny wakes feeling like death. It's an effort for him to get up. So! The day begins again. Can you realise what a strain this must be on Johnny's body? He is slowly destroying himself.

A body constantly under stress must respond to the stress; sooner or later the capacity to respond becomes exhausted, leaving the body over-stressed. In this condition the thymus gland which controls the body's immune system shrinks and has no effect on the white cells which defend the body against infection. With lowered defences disease is almost inevitable.

It is very hard for me to give you the solutions to your problems that you would love to hear. Nobody else can do that—only you! If you are stressed, lonely and downhearted, try some of the ideas I list below to help brighten up your life!

- ❖ Take a course at TAFE. Many TAFE colleges hold courses in such things as photography, languages, Chinese brush painting, computers, typing, accountancy, bridge, pottery, astrology, car maintenance, woodwork, floral art, interior design, leather work, tapestry, to mention but a few. Contact your local TAFE or evening college for more detailed information.
- ❖ Charity work gives you a feeling of being needed, also you are meeting people. Community work, hospital help, Meals on Wheels. Approach your local community centre and find out where they need help.
- ❖ Join a painting class. Take up bush walking. Join the local garden club or maybe the book club. Learn square or ballroom dancing. Take up a musical instrument.
- ❖ Join a social club. Most areas have branches of The Singles' Club, PWP (Parents Without Partners), BPW (Business and Professional Women), Toastmasters, Probus, The View Club, to name just a few. Consult your local newspaper or phone book; see which one suits you.
- ❖ If your interests are more artistic, join the Art Gallery Association, the National Heritage Society, ADFAS (Australian and Decorative Fine Arts Society), the Friends of the Historic Homes Society, the Botanical Garden Society or the Alliance Francaise.
- ❖ Study your atlas and plan an unusual holiday. You decide where you wish to go. Consult your travel agent for brochures and ideas.
- ❖ Take up a sport-choose from bowls, golf, tennis, squash, soccer, horse riding, sailing, wind surfing, surfing, netball, skiing, croquet, flying, hang gliding, gliding.
- ❖ By joining a club you will make new friends and become more outgoing. You won't be thinking about yourself and your problems as much. Playing a sport will give you a sense of achievement.
- ❖ A pet can be a great companion. I have two dogs, a poodle and a rottweiler. I love them dearly, they ask for nothing and give me so

much pleasure. Old people who look after their pets live longer than people the same age without pets. It gives them a will to live; they feel needed!

❖ Join a video club for hours of entertainment.
❖ Trace your family's history. Genealogy can be fun. Buy a book by Janet Reakes called *The A to Z Genealogical Handbook*.
❖ Learn a language. Find a teacher or buy some tapes.

Curing Loneliness

For the Girls

Treat yourself to some beauty therapy. Consult a hairdresser, have your hair tinted and restyled. Buy a stunning outfit, try a new perfume, something different. Many department stores offer a free make-up service and advice—why not try a new image? A different you! Visit the bookshop and buy the latest bestseller. Take time out, relax in a scented oil bath, along with a tall glass of chilled champagne.

Buy a high fashion magazine. There's one to suit all tastes, all age groups. Try *Harper's Bazaar, Studio, Taxi, She, Follow Me, Mode, Vogue, Dolly, Fashion*.

Read a book on how to improve your relationships or your sex life; a healthy sex life that gives you pleasure is an important part of feeling and looking great.

Self-help the Natural Way

Acupuncture, hypnosis, yoga, mountain spas, a holiday—anything that reduces stress and restores peace of mind is valuable.

Plato, a Greek philosopher who lived around 400BC, maintained even then that 'all the diseases of the body proceed from the mind and soul'.

Toning up the whole nervous system

Find the centre point of your forehead and in a one-centimetre radius as hard as you can for 30 seconds. Massaging this area will bring a sense of peace and tranquillity.

From the Health Food Store

Eleutherococcus is a substance derived from a plant called *Eleuthero-coccus senticosus*, which belongs to the same family of plants as gin-seng. It is referred to as a drug but acts like a tonic, countering the effects of stress and improving mental processes.

These all have a calming and soothing effect: L-Tryptophan (script only), Valerian herb, Passion flower, Skullcap, Ginseng and Royal jelly.

Drugs

Medical Drugs

Disease caused by medical treatment accounts for thousands of deaths each year. Apart from a great deal of suffering due to what doctors lightly refer to as side-effects, medical drugs of any kind can only in the long term cause damage. Let Dr Harris L. Coulter, Ph D, enlighten you:

> *Modern scientific medical practise relies very largely on medicines whose ultimate effect is to impair the patient's immune system. This is no secret, no great discovery. It is discussed in all the relevant literature. But it has never seemed significant until today when the world is faced with an epidemic rooted in a pervasive crippling of the immune system. The drugs synthesised since the end of World War II have achieved their end—the antibiotic sterilisation, more or less, of patient's bodies at the expense of the immune system, and AIDS is the last stop on the line. The immune system cannot be undermined indefinitely without a price being paid. The chickens have come home to roost.*

Dr Harris L. Coulter, *AIDS and Syphilis, the Hidden Link.*

Alcohol

1. Uses up vitamin B from the body.
2. Causes small red veins (broken capillaries) on nose and cheeks.
3. Dulls the brain.
4. Changes body metabolism
5. Makes it difficult to concentrate and can be addictive.
6. Will eventually destroy the brain and liver cells.

Nicotine

1. Affects the oxygen in the blood.
2. Affects the body cells.
3. Dulls the brain.
4. Causes wrinkles in the skin.
5. Takes vitamin C from the body (one cigarette destroys 25 mg of vitamin C).
6. Causes colds, emphysema, heart disease and lung cancer.

Marijuana

1. Destroys the brain cells (has been proven).
2. Decreases the sex drive (not at first but later).
3. Makes it difficult to concentrate.
4. Causes fits of deep depression.
5. Slows down bodily reactions.
6. Can eventually lead to irreversible schizophrenia.

Note: Drugs can destroy people's lives. Their use can lead to addiction to hard drugs like cocaine or heroin; it has been proven that all the so-called 'recreational' drugs are addictive and life destroying. Read James A. Mitchener's book *The Drifters*. Make sure your teenage children read it—they'll be off drugs for life!

How to Relax

Try using your mind to relax your body. There are several ways to do this, both at home and at the local community centre where yoga and relaxation classes are held. Look in your telephone directory under the heading Alternative Health Services (Yellow Pages) to help you with ideas.

Once again it is up to the individual. With outside courses you have the support of others plus the commitment of attending the class. Most people need group therapy support.

Home Relaxation

Relaxation is a necessity, not a luxury. Forget the housework, business chores or whatever; you deserve time for you to relax.

Now, how to relax? Play some soft music or relaxation tapes. Lie back in a comfortable armchair, feet up, eyes closed, relax all your muscles, beginning at your feet and working up to the top of your head, breathe deeply through your nose, breathe in and out—*relax*.

Concentrate on one word, a flower or a candle flickering, breathe in and out; continue for ten minutes or so. If your mind begins to wander, focus your attention back on the subject you are thinking about. Learn to programme your mind, to turn it off! This is so important.

Sleep

A good night's sleep is something everyone dreams of but your body's metabolism differs from time to time. Some nights you may go off to sleep as soon as your head hits the pillow, other nights you may lie awake for hours. This is natural; it depends on how tired you feel, how het up you are and what you have been doing during the day.

Try to get eight hours sleep a night. As we grow older we don't need as much sleep, in fact some people can survive on three hours and feel perfectly rested. Other people need ten hours; like everything else, it depends on the individual. Try not to eat a heavy fatty meal before going to bed, as your digestive system will have to work overtime and you will not sleep as well.

To help you sleep
- ❖ Make sure the windows are open and there is plenty of fresh air.
- ❖ Take a warm bath with herbs or scented oil, lie back, soak and relax.
- ❖ Play some soothing music.
- ❖ Use a herb pillow under your normal pillow.
- ❖ Make love.
- ❖ Chamomile tea does wonders.
- ❖ Take a glass of hot water with lemon juice and honey to bed.
- ❖ Run through the alphabet, A to Z, thinking of countries or flower titles beginning with each letter.
- ❖ Say your prayers.
- ❖ Don't take any sleeping tablets; these are addictive and dangerous. Use the home relaxation exercise above.
- ❖ Exercise helps. People who regularly exercise sleep better—but don't

exercise before going to bed.

❖ Before you go to sleep, run through all the nice positive things you have done that day, savour the pleasant things, smile at them and make yourself a promise that tomorrow will be even better. What made today a great day will work forever... SWEET DREAMS ...

When things go wrong
As they sometimes will,
When the road you're
Trudging seems all up hill,
When the funds are low
And the debts are high
And you want to smile
But you have to sigh,
When care is pressing
You down a bit,
Rest if you must but don't quit.

Life is queer with its
Twists and turns,
As everyone of us
Sometimes learns,
And many a failure
Turns about
When he might have won had he stuck it out;
Don't give up though
The pace seems slow—
You may succeed
With another blow.

Success is failure
Turned inside out—
The silver tint of the
Clouds of doubt,

RIGHT: A field of daylilies inviting you to float away stressful thoughts

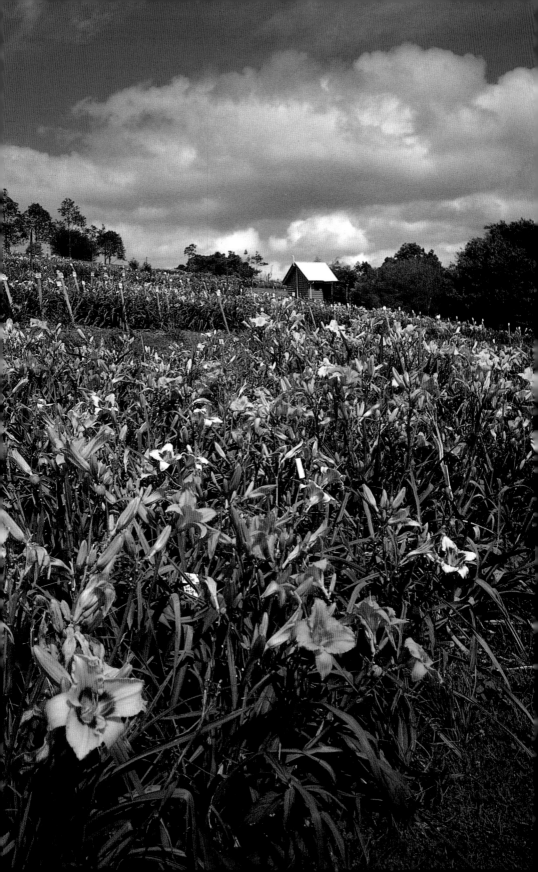

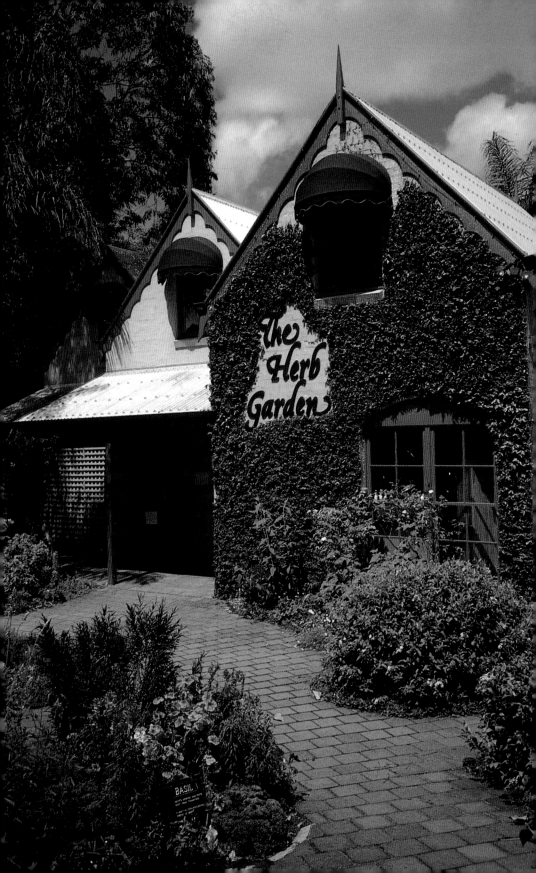

And you never can tell
How close you are,
It may be near
When it seems so far;
So stick to the fight
When you're hardest hit—
It's when things seem worst
That you must not quit.

Anon.

LEFT: *The Herb Cottage, Montville*

CHAPTER 4 # Beauty

Beauty comes from within but one can always enhance what nature has given by eating the correct foods, thereby eliminating pimples, acne, blemishes and clogged pores, and by following my overall programmme.

It doesn't matter if we are sixteen or sixty, it's never too late to pamper ourselves by applying a little paint to improve our self esteem. There is nothing more refreshing than looking into the mirror and seeing clear skin, shiny hair and sparkling eyes!

The woman who slops around in her dressing gown until noon with no makeup and unkempt hair certainly does not feel beautiful. It is essential at the beginning of each day to apply makeup and style your hair in preparation for a fun-filled day.

We would all love to look like our favourite star and we can, without spending a fortune, as you'll discover when you follow this chapter and learn some helpful tips on turning

YOU! INTO A STAR

Your Skin

Cleanse—tone—moisturise. A basic skin care routine using these three elements will contribute to making your skin look good at all times; regular cleansing helps skin to look fresh and glowing. Apply the cleanser and toner morning and night, using a moisturiser under your makeup in the morning and a night cream before going to bed. A daily skin routine is essential to maintain a healthy complexion, along with your diet and exercise programme.

The cleanser

Before going to bed use the cleanser to clean dirt and makeup from your face and neck. Thoroughly rub it into your skin and wash off with water. If you must use soap, make sure it is pure and not perfumed, as detergent-based soaps tend to remove oils from the skin. If you are unsure what type of cleanser to use for your skin type, consult a beauty sales assistant or your beautician. The same applies for the toner and moisturiser.

The toner

Toners remove all left-over cleanser and makeup residues from the skin. Use an alcohol-free toner (some astringent toners contain degrees of alcohol). Toning helps refine the skin pores and restores the pH balance, leaving a fresh soft skin.

The moisturiser

This is the most important step of the three. A moisturiser leaves a protective film on the skin surface, thus acting as a barrier against our environment—wind, sun, pollution and central heating. A moisturiser stops the skin from becoming too dry, thus avoiding wrinkles and ageing. Use a specially formulated eye cream for the delicate area around your eyes.

In the morning, before applying your make-up, cleanse and tone to remove all excess oil. Your skin should feel very soft. Next apply your moisturiser. If you wish you can now spray your face lightly with Evian water, so you have a fresh face on which to begin applying your foundation. DON'T FORGET: If you are spending time in the sun apply a sunscreen with SPF15+.

Before going to bed remove your makeup with the cleanser, followed by the toner, and then apply your night cream and eye cream.

Anti-ageing Products

The first and best anti-ageing product is a good diet.

Our skin begins the ageing process once we reach twenty. Consider some of the wonderful anti-ageing products on the market today and make an investment in your future face. Seek advice on what cream will best suit your skin type. Use it on both face and neck. Always apply an eye cream at night—the skin around the eyes is very fine and therefore ages quickly.

Makeup

The only person who can make up your face is you! Know your own face. What suits one person may not suit another. It is important to develop your own look.

Take your time. Apply everything carefully to achieve a subtle look, making sure your face looks healthy and natural. Night makeup can be more dramatic. Treat your face as a canvas, yourself as an artist; learn by your mistakes until you have everything *perfect*!

Before you begin it is important to arrange the best lighting possible. Any room with artificial light will do. Natural daylight is the most difficult to work with, as it casts shadows on your face (put your back to the window). A three-way mirror with tiny light bulbs around it in a windowless room is ideal.

Makeup Requirements

Headband (to keep makeup off hair)
Soft brush (sable) for powder
Sponge for foundation
Soft brush for blusher
Lipstick brush
Small comb and brush for eyelashes and brows
Stick for eyeshadow
Eyelash curler
Cottonwool balls and buds
Concealer for blemishes
Foundation
Powder
Blusher
Lipsticks
Lip gloss
Eyeshadow
Eyeliner
Eyebrow pencil
Mascara
Compact (compressed powder)

Tips

Eye and lip pencils: To keep a good point after sharpening, put in the fridge for fifteen minutes. Allow them to return to normal temperature before using.

Mascara: If a new mascara is too runny remove the lid for a couple of days to let it dry out. To dry mascara fast between coats, use your hairdryer.

Always keep sponges and brushes clean.

Applying Makeup

1. Moisturiser.
2. Concealer: Concealers can be used to hide blemishes, red cheeks and dark circles under the eyes. I prefer a liquid concealer as it tends to give a more natural appearance; a stick concealer can pull the skin and leave a harsh line.
3. Foundation: Find out what type of foundation suits your skin. Many women make the mistake of trying to conceal their age with a thick foundation, but this only emphasises lines and wrinkles. When you shop for the right foundation, test it on your cheek, not on the back of your hand; the skin there is not the same. If you apply the foundation in the direction of facial hair growth it will be smooth on the skin. Always take foundation down to your neck to avoid making a sharp jaw line. Let your face dry before applying powder.
4. Powder: When your foundation has completely set, use a cotton ball to dab on translucent powder, then brush off excess powder with a makeup brush, working downwards to flatten facial hairs. If you want a healthy look use a brownish blush on your cheekbones and forehead.
5. Blusher: Blusher will certainly light up your face. For a natural look powdered blusher is best. Apply gently with a soft brush along your cheekbone, finishing where the outer eye area ends. Do not dab big blotches on your cheeks—you will end up looking like a kewpie doll.
6. Eye makeup: See next section.
7. Lip makeup: See page 56.

Your Eyes

Tips for puffiness around the eyes

- ❖ Cold tea bags, one on each eye.
- ❖ Cotton balls soaked in cold milk, one on each eye.
- ❖ Place a slice of cucumber on each eye.
- ❖ Lie down for ten minutes on a flat surface—this should brighten your eyes.
- ❖ After a face cleanse, apply Vita cream under the eyes.
- ❖ Remove eye makeup with an eye cream or any natural oil such as olive or coconut.

To make up the eyes

Apply foundation to the eye area, brush lightly with powder, brush eyeshadow up to brows, use eyeliner to shape eyes, apply mascara, and groom eyebrows following the tips below.

Eyeshadow

Use eyeshadows in subtle colours. Please, no more bright blue! A soft beige, a golden or a charcoal; brush it up into the brows. All other makeup should be kept low-key too. If you extend eyeshadow beyond the outer corner of the eyes, remember to extend your eyebrows too.

Eyeliner

One can achieve so much with an eyeliner pencil; if you prefer you can use a liquid eyeliner but make sure you have a steady hand. A dark liner tends to shrink the eyes. To open up your eyes, run a white kohl liner above the lower lashes. With a liner you can alter the shape of your eyes, make small eyes look larger, turn round eyes into doe eyes and so on—try some experiments. A grey or beige liner gives a softer look. Black can look very heavy.

Eyebrows

It is best to pluck eyebrows after a bath or shower. Use a touch of Vaseline over the area; this way the plucking won't hurt as much. Pluck from underneath the hair and shape from below the brow; tweezer straggly hairs on top. If you need to shape your brows, use a very sharp eyebrow pencil and draw in tiny feathery strokes to resemble small hairs. Don't draw the whole eyebrow in one heavy arched stroke.

Use a grey or charcoal pencil; black is too harsh. Brush over the pencil with a small eye brush. To keep the brows in shape add a touch of Vaseline, gel or clear lip gloss. If your brows are heavy or black, have them bleached (by a professional at first); don't experiment on yourself. The same applies if your brows are fair and you wish to have them dyed darker.

Mascara

In general, mascara looks better black. If you are a blonde, however, you may choose brown, navy or grey. Apply three layers, making sure each coat dries before applying the next. If you are in a hurry, dry with your hairdryer.

Don't let the lashes clog together. Once the mascara is dry use an eyelash curler. Hold the curler to the lash for the count of 50 then let go, brush with a small comb and apply the eyelash curler again. Always mascara both top and lower lashes; so many women neglect their lower lashes, then wonder why their eyes look unfinished. For a wonderful evening effect, use black mascara, then tip the ends with gold or silver. If your lashes are short you could experiment with false lashes—why not?

SMILE

A smile costs nothing, but creates much!
It enriches those who receive it, without impoverishing those who give
*   it away.*
It happens in a flash and yet the memory of it lasts forever.
None are so rich they can get along without it
And none so poor that they cannot be made rich.
Fosters goodwill in a business, and is the countersign of friends ....
It is rest to weary, daylight to the discouraged, sunshine to the sad,
and nature's best antidote for trouble.
Yet it cannot be bought, begged or borrowed, or stolen, for it is of no
worth to anyone until it is given away.
If someone is too tired to give you a smile give them one of yours ...
For no-one needs a smile as much as someone who has no more to
give!

Anon.

55

Your Lips

That winning smile

Shy of smiling? There is no need to be. If your teeth embarrass you, visit your dentist, who will give you good advice on crowns, bridges, straightening, tooth care in general. Your six-monthly check should include a thorough clean.

Always carry a traveller's fold-up toothbrush and tooth floss in your bag, plus a mouth freshener.

Brush your gums as well as your teeth after every meal and run floss between your teeth. Throw out your old toothbrush every two or three months.

Vaseline rubbed lightly on teeth can give a shiny effect.

When choosing a lipstick be sure it enhances your tooth colour. Try out a new lipstick by smiling in front of the mirror. A bright red lipstick will make your teeth look whiter. Wear pinks, corals and beiges if your teeth tend to be a little yellow.

Requirements for the perfect mouth

Four lipsticks (no more, who needs clutter?):
    Deep glowing red for evening
    Brownish pink
    Lightish pink (not too pale)
    Bronze orange
Lip brush for applying lipstick
Lip pencil
Lip gloss

For a long-lasting result when applying lipstick, start with foundation, brush lightly with powder, outline lips with a sharp lip pencil, apply lipstick with a lip brush, and finish with lip gloss.

Lip Makeup

Full lips: Outline with a brownish pencil just inside the natural lip shade. With tiny strokes define the centre of the lips. Colour in with lipstick. Use a non-gloss lipstick as this will make the lips look less full.
Thin lips : Use lip pencil just outside natural lip area. Colour over this

line with coloured lipstick. For a more subtle effect blot a deep colour and apply lip gloss. If your lower lip is thin, make it fuller by lining with brownish pencil just outside the lips and line very slightly at the upper lip corners. Cover with lipstick.

Wrinkled lips: Stretch lips gently with finger and thumb and outline with a skin-toned pencil. This helps prevent lipstick running outside the lip line. Release lips and brush with lipstick.

Lip bleed: Apply a coat of pale concealer to the lips and set with dusting powder; outline using a lip pencil the same shade as your lipstick. Fill in colour and stop just inside pencil line.

Chapped lips: To prevent lips chapping wear a sun block SPF15+, and natural coloured zinc cream. Apply Nyal's Lipeeze or a similar cream.

An application of lip cream before going to bed can give lips a fuller, plumper appearance the next day, and discourage lipstick from bleeding into fine lines.

Lip base helps lipstick to slide on smoothly, and then sets lip colour. It reduces lipstick smearing and feathering even after eating and drinking.

Your Hair

You can be wearing the best dress in the world, but if your hair doesn't look good, you won't look good!

YOUR HAIR IS YOUR
GREATEST BEAUTY ACCESSORY

Have you changed your style in the last ten years? If not, it's time you did!

Find yourself an excellent hairstylist (ask around or look for someone with a smart style and ask them the name of their hairdresser). Remember that what looks good on a movie star, a model or your friend may not look good on you. Browse through some magazines and pick a style that you feel will suit you.

Don't let the hairdresser cut off too much hair all at once, but take off a little at a time. Choose an appointment on a weekday, not on Thursday night or Saturday morning as these are busy days and you won't get all the attention you require. Near shoulder length, about level with your chin, is the most feminine, versatile and flattering. In the daytime one can wear it in a bob, fluffed out, curly perm, ponytail. In the evening it can be styled on top of the head, some hair up, some down or pushed to the side with a fancy comb.

You will find a wide variety of hair accessories on the market—scrunchies, ribbons, clips, combs, flowers. Shop around.

Make sure the style you choose will suit your lifestyle, that you feel comfortable with it, and that you can manage it yourself.

For a full bouffant look, when blowdrying your hair lean your head over to look at the floor and scrunch the hair towards your forehead.

Colouring your hair: If you must colour your hair yourself and it's the first time, test the colour on a few strands to make sure it's right for you. I strongly recommend going to a professional hair colourist who will know exactly what colour will suit you, how long to leave it on, whether you need a tint or semi-permanent colour. Once you are familiar with the procedure then go ahead and do it yourself!

There is no excuse for not having your hair looking good, not with all the gels, mousses, hairsprays, blowdryers, curling wands, heated rollers and brushes available. With a little time and patience your hair will become your crowning glory.

Shampooing

Wet hair thoroughly, apply a small amount of shampoo to the palm of your hand, add a little water to the shampoo to dilute it, then apply to hair and massage very carefully. Don't rub hard as this can break your hair. Apply a conditioner after washing, leave on for a couple of minutes then rinse off. Pat excess water from hair, comb with a widetoothed comb. If your hair is dry leave the conditioner on for a longer time and use a weekly treatment.

Don't wash your hair every day, as it will lose its natural oils. About three or four times weekly is sufficient.

Fine hair: Needs to be washed at least every second day. Alternate shampoo brands and remember perms can be disastrous for fine hair! Keep it short and sleek and full and fluffy. Use a diffuser on your hairdryer.

Medium hair: It does not need much shampooing, but can take two or more washes weekly. Lucky the ones with this kind of hair, it will go anywhere.

Oily hair: Keep it washed and clean. Oily hair needs the most washing, but remember if washed too often the scalp is stimulated thus producing more oil. Do not use cream rinse conditioner on oily hair and don't eat fatty foods.

Coarse hair: Give yourself a weekly treatment. Keep this type of hair to a medium to long length with a good cut. If it is too long it will become heavy and lose its style.

The best way to dry hair is naturally. Electrical appliances such as blow dryers, curling wands and electric rollers are the worst of all for drying, breaking or weakening hair. Remember when blow drying don't use on HOT. Try always to towel dry first to lessen the time with a blow dryer.

If you colour your hair it is best to condition it only once a week, as conditioner removes colour.

Never use soap or detergent-based shampoo on hair as they make it dull.

The essential ingredients for beautiful shining hair are exercise, fresh fruit and vegetables, iron, plenty of rain water, vitamin B and most of all no fatty junk foods!

Tips

* Use natural fibre brushes on your hair. Bristle is better than nylon, wire or metal, which tend to break your hair.
* When you judge a style a full length mirror is a must.
* Change your hair shampoo and conditioner every so often. Your hair can become accustomed to one brand and lose its lustre.
* To make hair blonder, squeeze and strain a lemon into cool water, apply to hair, leave for ten minutes, rinse off.
* Don't have a perm done more than twice a year. Perms and tints are very drying to the hair. Take time and use the blowdryer or rollers.
* If you are going grey, don't tint your hair very dark brown or black— this shows every line and wrinkle. Keep to the pale browns, ash blonde and beige shades.

❖ Wet hair breaks easily. If you pull at a wet tangle the hair will break. It's also best not to brush your hair when wet; comb through gently with a wide-toothed comb instead.

Your Hands

Hands can tell it all! I should look after mine a lot better than I do. I spend too much time in the garden and often forget my gloves. Don't let this happen to you!

Always keep a tube of handcream near basins and sinks and use it each time you wash up, whatever. Take note: Don't use very hot water when washing up; this makes hands perspire and can cause dermatitis.

Use lined rubber gloves when gardening or doing similar work. Apply hand cream first, then put on your gloves. If you don't like gloves, rub your nails through a cake of soap; this will keep the dirt out.

To keep your hands soft, mix lemon juice and sugar together, rub into hands, leave ten minutes and rinse off.

If your hands are chapped, soak them in warm milk for about ten minutes, rinse off. Repeat daily till they are better. Wear gloves in cold weather to prevent chapping.

Nails

Nails grow about 6 mm a month. It takes about six months to grow a normal nail. Scissors or clippers can cause nails to break or split. Always use an emery board to file your nails (never a steel nail file). File from the sides to the middle of the nail, always working in one direction, never sawing backwards and forwards. If one nail breaks, file the others down to match, otherwise your nails will look untidy. When selecting a nail polish remover buy an oil-based one as acetone is very drying. Use a cuticle cream to soften the cuticles (Vaseline is just as good). There are several good nail hardeners on the market— I think Herome is excellent.

Tools for the manicure:
Nail brush
Emery boards
Cuticle cream

Orange sticks
Oily nail polish remover
Nail polish base
Hand lotion
Bowl of water
Towel
Favourite nail polish

Manicure: If you are wearing nail polish, file your nails with the old polish on as it will help to protect them. Remove polish with cotton wool soaked in remover. Soak nails in soapy water, then dry. Rub cuticle cream into cuticles, pushing them back with an orange stick or a cotton bud. Wash nails again ready to polish. Paint on base coat, let dry. Paint on two coats of nail polish, drying after each coat or you may have to begin again. If you are in a hurry dip your finger tips in a basin of cold water or use your hairdryer.
Note: A base coat protects the nails from dyes in the polish. A top coat protects the polish and adds lustre.

Your Feet

Buy the best soft leather, medium heeled shoes you can afford—this is a necessity! Don't stagger around in cheap high-heeled shoes all day; they will ruin your feet. Your feet swell during the day so it's best to shop for shoes in the afternoon. If you intend travelling some distance by aeroplane make sure your shoes are a size larger than usual as your feet always swell! Use a foot deodorant if your feet have a tendency to be niffy. If you have corns or calluses see a chiropodist. Try to walk around barefoot as nature intended, for the earth sends electrical charges through the soles of your feet up through your body. When cutting toenails, cut straight across; if you shape them into the corners you could develop ingrown toenails.

Always keep your feet as dry as possible as perspiration and dampness cause tinea which can take months to heal. When painting toenails choose a pale pink polish or use natural. If you must wear thongs, please, only on the beach ...

Pedicure: Soak feet in soapy water (you can use shampoo) for ten minutes. Rub a cake of soap across your toenails and scrub hard with a nail brush after soaking; your toenails will be softened and easier to cut. Use a pumice stone or a foot file on heels and soles. Pat feet dry, rub cuticle cream into nails and push cuticles back with an orange stick. Make sure your nails are thoroughly clean, separate your toes with cotton wool and apply nail polish.

The Weekly Facial

If you can afford a facial from a beautician, I would recommend having one monthly. They are extremely beneficial and relaxing.

Do-it-yourself facial

1. Cleanse
2. Tone
3. Exfoliate
4. Face steam
5. Mask

Cleanse and tone the skin as outlined on page 50. Next use an exfoliating mask. Leave it on for ten minutes before rubbing it off with the fingertips; this peels off the dead skin cells and reveals the fresher skin underneath.

Next fill a bowl or handbasin with boiling water. Position your cleansed face above the bowl, cover your head with a towel, making sure the steam doesn't escape, and steam your face for five minutes. This helps to open the pores, which will allow the face mask to penetrate to the active layers of the skin. Apply the face mask, leave on for twenty minutes and wash off. Tweeze your brows while the mask is setting.

For the greatest benefit, choose a facial mask which suits your skin's needs: deep cleansing, pore refining, hydrating. Find out from a trained beautician which one suits your skin type best.

You can make your own mask with cornflour mixed with water to form a paste; apply a thin layer to your face and when dry wash off with a face washer. Beaten egg whites make a good mask.

The Bath

People have been making a ritual of bathing for generations. The Aegeans were the first civilisation to provide bathrooms. Bathing occupied an important place in the lives of the Greeks too.

In Finland men and women took steam baths together. They would beat their skin with twigs to stimulate circulation and cleanse the skin, completing the process by plunging into a steam spa, then rolling in the snow.

In China and Japan the bath is usually made of wood; it is a considerable size and filled with very hot water. The entire family may soak in the tub, but they cleanse and rinse themselves thoroughly before they get into the bath. Massage is often associated with bathing in Asia.

The Romans, with their love of luxury, would undress, anoint themselves with oil, indulge in violent exercise, after which they would proceed to a hot room, then a warm one, followed by a cold bath; the body would once more be anointed and the process completed.

Russians and Eastern Europeans have a great love for hot steam baths, resulting in a multitude of bath houses. These simply consist of a steam room and a cold bath.

You too can enjoy a luxury bath followed by a cold shower in your own home.

What you will need
Radio or tape player
Bath oil
Cake of scented soap
Pumice stone
Nail brush
Razor
Loofah
Facial peel and mask
Body oil or lotion
Talcum powder
Soft fluffy towel

Add to your running bath water your favourite oil or bubble bath, salts, or fresh herbs from the garden such as crushed mint, thyme or lavender, or even milk. These help soften the skin. While the water is running, give yourself a facial and leave the face mask on. Now turn on some soothing music and plunge into the bath water. Scrub yourself all over with the loofah; this works on cellulite (tiny dimples in the skin) and stimulates the lymph system. Use the pumice stone on your heels, the soles of your feet and your elbows—wherever you feel roughness. Brush your nails and push back the cuticles. Shave your legs and under your arms. Lie back and relax for a while, then wash your mask off with the washer. When you get out you can take a quick cold shower if you like (it is up to you). Dry yourself with a towel, smooth body lotion all over your skin and dust yourself with talc powder. Put on your favourite glamorous house gown, then give yourself a manicure and pedicure. Curl up with a good book, a cup of tea and take time out for an hour or two.

ONE NEEDS TO PAMPER ONESELF!

Sun Tanning

Always wear a sunscreen when outdoors. With the depleting ozone layer and Australia already claiming the highest rate of skin cancer in the world, statistics say that two out of every three Australians will develop skin cancer. It is sheer suicide to go without some protection. The summer months are high risk months for sunburn, but you can get burned *any time of the year.*

Wear a hat with a large brim outdoors; it will reduce the ultraviolet radiation reaching your face by up to 50 per cent.

Slip! Slop! Slap! We've all been bombarded by this slogan, but are we taking it seriously? It's vital that we do! Avoid sunlight exposure by slipping on a T-shirt, slopping on some sunscreen and slapping on a hat!

You can achieve a healthy tan by applying a sunscreen SPF15+ to your face and a sun lotion between SPF4 and SPF12 (depending on your skin type) all over your body when you are at the beach. Remember that sunscreen doesn't last all day—reapply as often as the directions say.

RIGHT: *Well cared for glossy hair*

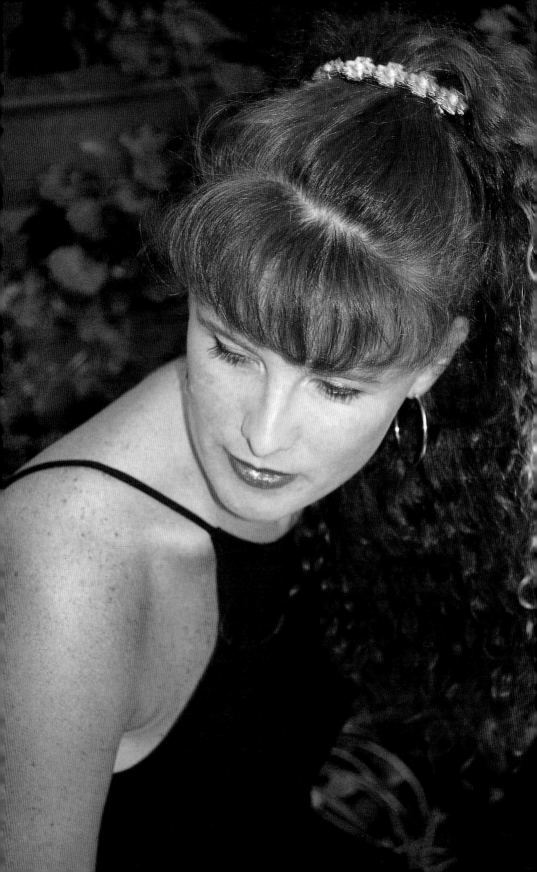

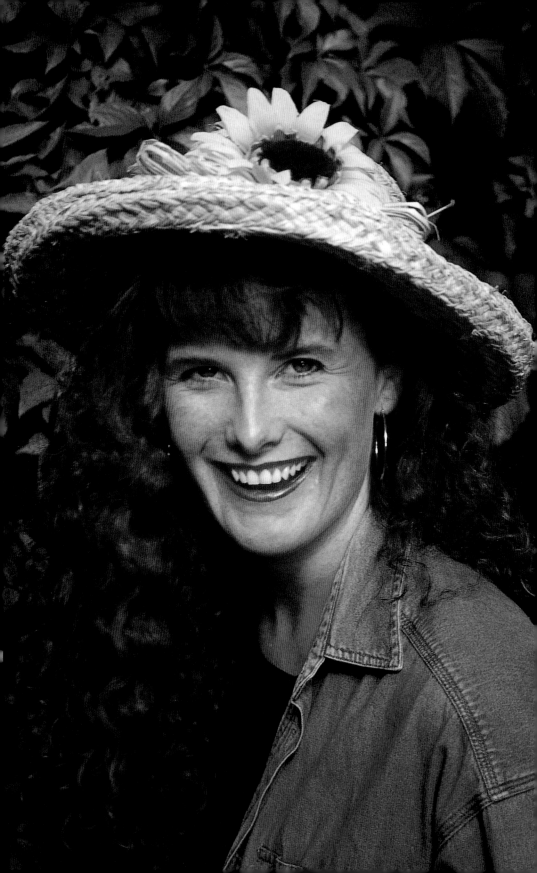

After a day's outing at the beach apply after-sun lotion after your shower to replace the moisture lost from your skin during the day.

Babies and tiny tots should not have their bodies covered in sunscreen as their skin is more likely to absorb the chemicals in sunscreens. Use a small amount of SPF15+ on baby's face, hands and feet and cover them up. The Cancer Council's sun protection suits are great value.

The higher you go up into the mountains the greater the risk of sunburn. UV radiation increases by about 15 per cent every 1000 metres above sea level.

Skin cancers

Watch for spots. Early detection can result in a cure for about 90 per cent of skin cancers. Be alert if a spot or mole changes in size, shape or colour! Early skin cancers are rarely painful.

Deportment and Posture

It is a fact that hunched shoulders and a slumped body posture actually make a depressed person feel more defeated and depressed.

If you hunch your back, practice walking with a book on your head for ten minutes a day. Never forget the book is there—remember, head up, like a puppet on a string, shoulders back, stomach pulled in, buttocks held tightly together and the spine straight.

When sitting up, hold your head high and never slouch, especially over a dinner table. There should be no gap between your spine and the back of your chair. Never sit with your legs apart as it looks most unattractive, but don't cross your legs either, as this can cut circulation. Cross your feet at the ankles or put both legs to one side with your feet together.

FOLLOW THIS CHAPTER TO THE LETTER AND
YOU WILL 'TURN INTO A STAR'

LEFT: *Happiness is a smile*

Hormone Replacement Therapy (HRT)

The human body when in good health is as robust and durable as that of any other member of the animal world. Unfortunately, however, due to the various bad habits—mainly dietary bad habits—that civilised humans have managed to invent, the people who indulge in them sooner or later show the evidence of wear and tear in the form of various health problems.

The worst of the many harmful substances contained in our traditional Western diet is fat, and whereas nutritionists all agree that ideally fat in the diet should not exceed 10% of the total energy value (kilojoules) in the diet, the typical modern diet contains about 40%. It is this intake of fat which is the prime cause of most of the 'diseases of civilisation', the major ones being heart disease and other circulatory problems, cancer, arthritis, asthma, migraine, pre-menstrual tension, diabetes, prostate and menopausal problems. Regardless of what doctors believe about heredity and the unavoidability of these problems, it is a simple matter to arrest and, in most cases, reverse these ailments simply by strict dietary correction. And very quickly too, as I have explained at length in my several books.

Estrogen and progesterone are the female sex hormones and their production in the body is influenced by the level of fat in the diet. It is the highly excessive level of fat in the modern diet compared with the simpler diets of many years ago that causes the abnormal production of these hormones and premature sexual development of females, and their larger bosoms, that occurs today. Whereas in years past girls began to menstruate at age about sixteen, today they begin at about twelve.

It is the excess fat that is also responsible for the almost universal weight problems of today with the accompanying increased risk of every disease in the book including cancer, particularly breast cancer, which is strongly influenced by hormone levels. Another problem more prevalent among women today is osteoporosis, the weakening of bones by their loss of calcium, supposedly caused by the lowered production of estrogen that occurs with menopause.

It is also this lack of estrogen that is held responsible for the other distressing symptoms that occur at menopause such as hot flushes, night sweats, mental problems, sleeplessness, bladder problems and the increased danger of blood clots and heart attacks, and it has been shown that hormone replacement therapy (HRT) may help to relieve some of these symptoms. For this reason the therapy is becoming widely used.

But—

Many medical research doctors are extremely suspicious of hormone replacement therapy because there are too many inconsistencies and conflicting data about it as well as evidence that shows HRT results in a significantly increased risk of cancer. And whereas HRT supposedly protects against osteoporosis, it has been pointed out (New Scientist, Oct. 23, 1993) that hip fracture from osteoporosis is just as common among men as it is in women, having increased threefold in the last thirty years. Moreover it is a fact that the lowest incidence of heart disease occurs in countries where women's estrogen levels are the lowest, as it is also with cancer.

What follows is hard to believe, but true—it has been proposed by some medical scientists that in order to prevent breast cancer, pre-menopausal women be routinely treated with a drug, GnRH, which affects the pituitary gland so to prevent the production of estrogen and progesterone. And then, because this results in menopausal effects in young women, they are given a certain amount of artificial estrogen replacement therapy to prevent these effects, and a course of synthetic progesterone every fourth month to ensure their continued fertility, which means they only have menstrual periods three times a year! On a trial of this 'preventive therapy', women on the GnRH treatment experienced severe osteoporosis, losing 2% of their bone mass in less than a year!

Another similar trial, a ten year one by the US Federal Government National Cancer Institute, involving 16 000 supposedly healthy women over age 35, has been in progress since early 1992. This trial, called the Breast Cancer Prevention Trial, is designed to determine whether the drug Tamoxifen effectively prevents the disease. $70 million has been allocated to this trial on the flimsy evidence that out of eight previous studies only one suggested any benefit could accrue to pre-menopausal women while at the same time another study showed that cancer risk was actually increased by the drug. To make things worse, it is already known that Tamoxifen causes a sevenfold increase in the incidence of blood clots, and increases the risk of endometrial cancer as much as five times, but the director of the trial says that this risk is no greater than it would be on estrogen therapy, but he did not add that endometrial cancer caused by Tamoxifen was much deadlier, causing liver damage as well.

In Britain most of the women who submit to HRT discontinue it, according to Guy's Hospital in London, the reasons being bleeding, feeling bloated, weight gain, nausea, breast tenderness and headaches, as well as *concern about cancer and effects as yet unknown.*

By now you are probably slowly shaking your head in wonderment at the absurd behaviour of supposedly intelligent people and you no doubt would shake all over if you knew of the complicity between various 'custodians of public health' and the pharmaceutical companies whose marketing methods make the cigarette companies look like amateurs and whose legal drugs cause more harm than all the illegal ones put together.

The alternative to hormone replacement therapy is to get healthy and fit and then throw all your medicines into the sea, whereupon, as Doctor Oliver Wendell Holmes once said, 'It would be so much better for man, and so much the worse for the fishes.'

Ross Horne

CHAPTER 5 Happiness

Oh, to be Happy!

Probably the biggest health problem in Australia and other Western countries is

UNHAPPINESS OR DEPRESSION

Unhappiness in the dictionary means 'not bringing or enjoying good fortune, sadness'.

Unhappy people wallow in self pity, they are depressed and moody, they worry and procrastinate. They are jealous of other's efforts, they criticise and intimidate others to try to make themselves feel better. They are consumed by anger, resentment and guilt and live in fear.

Happiness makes the world go round

Happiness in the dictionary means 'content' or 'satisfied'. To me:
Happiness is having a sense of self
Happiness is talent
Happiness is feeling good
Happiness is looking great
Happiness is giving
Happiness is peace
Happiness is laughter
Happiness is people, places and events
Happiness is fun
Happiness is responsibility
Happiness is creating
Happiness is self respect

Happiness is involvement
Happiness is being positive
Happiness is loving yourself and others
Happiness is playing childish games
Happiness is unselfishness
Happiness is unafraid of feeling
Happiness is fulfilment of life
Happiness is goal
Happiness is success
Happiness is taking time out to smell the roses

Happiness is like a butterfly.
The more you chase it, the more it will elude you,
but if you turn your attention to other things
it comes and softly sits on your shoulder.

Anon.

If life were a game, the happy people would be the players, the unhappy people the spectators. If life were a parade, the happy people would be standing on the sidewalk watching the parade go by. Happy people are active and involved. It is necessary to continually risk new activities, experiences, and people in order to be happy. Am I waiting for the phone to ring? Am I living life OR is life living me? ... ARE YOU HAPPY?

Dennis Wholey

I truly believe that the happiest people are those who love many things with passion. The key is loving intensely and loving many many things. Genius often comes from focusing on one thing, but geniuses are often unhappy people. Happy people have a wider focus. They love children and family and trees and cooking and eating and celebrating. They love sunrises and sunsets and snow and spring and winter and fall. They love life. They have even learned to love pain and despair, recognising that we must not dichotomise. We must not set up things like joy being the opposite of despair. It's just the other side of despair. These things are really one and the same thing and one often grows out of the other. Some of the greatest wisdom I've ever gained was from a despairing situation ...

Leo F. Buscaglia, Ph.D.

Have you ever noticed when you are feeling good about yourself other people become nice? Isn't it funny how they change!

The world is a reflection of ourselves. When we hate ourselves, we hate everybody else. When we love being who we are, the rest of the world is wonderful.

Andrew Matthews, *Being Happy*

The Key is the Mind

You may ask: 'But how can I be happy?'

The idea is to programme your mind.

When I first met my husband Ross Horne twenty years ago, I would often say to him, 'The mind controls the body.' When Ross wrote *The Health Revolution*, he gave me one of the first copies and in the front cover he wrote:

The mind controls the body, you've often told me that.
But both will work much better if you jog and lay off fat—
Look into the future, for some it's misery and strife ...
Take this advice and heed it—
You only have one life!

The first part of this book hopefully will help you sort out your diet and exercise programme and beauty routine. Now, how to make you feel happy and content. You have to talk yourself out of feeling lonely, despondent and depressed. Train your mind not to think too hard about your worries. Pull down the blind, as Scarlett O'Hara did in *Gone With the Wind*. She said, 'I'll think about that tomorrow!'

Unhappiness will kill you. Imagine your body a bag of living cells, tiny animals all forming communities. The liver cells, breast cells, lung cells and so on—they all want to live in harmony and in the right environment to function properly. The blood has to be kept nice and clean and free flowing. If you suffer from unhappiness your cells suffer too. As I mentioned in the stress chapter, the hormones release a chemical poison into your bloodstream and in the end you will become sick. It is vital to be as happy as you can.

Try to love yourself better. Think when you look in the mirror each day, 'I look great, I feel great and I am going to have a great day!' You'll find people will like you and your family and friends will benefit from your happy mood.

There are some wonderful books you can read on the power of the mind and on happiness. I have read several books on cancer cure. One book in particular impressed me greatly. Mrs X wrote, 'How I cured my cancer... I imagined the good cells like policemen rounding up the bad cells [cancer] and destroying them. Gobbling them up! I imagined the tumour becoming smaller and smaller and finally it went away.'

The placebo effect is a mind-blowing thing. A doctor wrote about some of his patients who suffered from various ills. He rolled some moist bread into small balls, painted them various colours to resemble pills and prescribed them to his hypochondriac patients, telling them to take a different coloured pill with each meal. The pills had a remarkable effect and the patients returned to tell him how much better they felt.

In his book *Getting Well Again* (1978), Dr Carl Simonton described dramatic remissions of cancer in patients; he had taught them to visualise the white cells of their immune systems as an army attacking their cancer cells and destroying them. Dr Simonton said, 'You are more in charge of your life—and even the development and progress of a disease, such as cancer—than you may realise. You may actually, through a power within you, be able to decide whether you live or die.'

CANCER IS A WORD, NOT A SENTENCE

In *Anatomy of an Illness* Norman Cousins tells of a meeting he had in Africa with Dr Albert Schweitzer, musician, physician and Nobel Prize winner. Replying to Cousins' question as to how the African tribal witchdoctors achieved such good results, Dr Schweitzer replied: 'It's supposed to be a professional secret, but I'll tell you anyway. The witchdoctor succeeds for the same reason all the rest of us succeed. Each patient carries his own doctor inside him. They come to us not knowing the truth. We are at our best, when we give the doctor who resides within each patient a chance to go to work.' (Lesson 1 for all medical students.)

The mind is a mysterious thing. There are mystic powers of the mind which we don't fully understand, such as hypnosis, levitation, ESP, clairvoyancy and mental telepathy. In this scientific world not much attention is paid to the aspects of the mind—we are too concerned with technology—but some pre-industrialised peoples possess powers of observation and thought transmission that are astonishing to us.

My father told me this story a long time ago: The year was 1929. My dad and his mate rode a Harley-Davidson motorbike and sidecar on an adventure trip around Australia. (They hold the record for the first motorbike and sidecar to go around Australia and are in the Guinness Book of Records.) The roads in those days were barely tracks; in fact, Robinson's, the Sydney map company, paid them £5 to map the road from Katherine to Darwin.

At night when they were settled in their sleeping bags under the stars, the Aborigines would creep out from the surrounding bush to look and touch their bike. Next day they would continue on their journey. Sometimes the country they traversed was so rough they could only travel a few miles, other days they would ride one hundred, but always the Aborigines would be waiting for their arrival, knowing they were coming—mental telepathy. Mrs Aeneas Gunn in her book *We of the Never Never* called it 'the Bush Telegraph' (means of communication by telepathy).

Many of us who live in modern industrialised societies have lost this sense, along with many other senses too. The point is:

IF YOU DON'T USE IT
YOU LOSE IT!

One can't expect to be happy and contented all the time. We all have our good and bad days. Fortunately I am a happy person and I try very hard to make all around me happy too. That is why I'm writing this book.

There was a day when I felt worried and depressed. I have rarely had this feeling in my life, but I had it then. A friend of mine visited and when I mentioned how down I felt, he suggested, 'Tomorrow we will go on a picnic and you'll forget all your problems!'

Next day we set off for West Head. What a wonderful day! We walked through Sydney's beautiful bushland. I had packed a delicious picnic lunch, which we enjoyed overlooking a picturesque beach. We talked and joked and when I returned home I felt terrific, a new person.

Happiness had returned; it just took that little bit of getting out of my own way.

No-one can constantly make you happy; they can help, but it's all up to you. If you are unhappy and not in a good state of mind the butterfly will elude you.

Three simple rules

1. We must like and love ourselves.

2. We must like others.

3. We must play and have fun doing childish and simple things. We should have a deep feeling of adventure, like young children at play. When people say they are unhappy, they have lost their love and joy of childlike play.

A Recreation Programme

'All work and no play makes one heck of a day.'

One must have a recreation programme to be happy

Johnny and Tommy work in the same dirty, noisy factory. Their jobs are monotonous.

Johnny (we've met him before) is unhappy. He has no recreation programme. He hates the job, he takes sick days off because he is depressed; when he is at work, he can't wait to leave to join his mates at the local pub. He drinks far too much and constantly arrives home late for dinner.

His wife is upset with their lifestyle and nags him. This makes him stay out more and the situation becomes worse.

On the weekend he is apathetic and worn out from apathy and drinking. He lounges around the house watching sport on TV and drinking. Monday comes and the vicious circle begins all over again. If Johnny doesn't change his ways and adopt some form of recreation programme, there is trouble ahead for the family.

If Johnny can't help himself with his habits, maybe his wife could call Al-Anon; they can help her with his problem!

Now we will take Tommy. He makes the most of the job. He feels content and happy. Why? Because he has a recreation programme! Instead of going to the pub each afternoon, he visits the local gym. He and his wife play tennis during the week and they have their friends from the club over for barbecues.

Tommy surfs on some weekends and takes his family along also. His surfing interest gives him pleasure and he looks forward to the new surfing magazines.

He takes his family on a holiday each year. They all enjoy a good relationship and a happy recreation programme.

I am endeavouring to point out just how important a recreation programme is to make you happy. Don't forget! It's not all work—one needs play as well. Sit down and take a good look at your present situation. If it's going nowhere, do something about it!

Programme Your Subconscious Mind

Learn to programme into your subconscious mind your aims, your goals, your projects, whether it be your health, money, a job, winning, succeeding, whatever. Tell yourself over and over again

I'LL MAKE IT
I WILL SUCCEED!

and you will through sheer determination and persistence.

> *Nothing in the world can take the place of persistence. Talent will not; nothing is more common than unsuccessful men with talent. Genius will not; unrewarded genius is almost a proverb. Education will not; the world is full of educated derelicts.*
>
> *Persistence and determination alone are omnipotent. The slogan 'Press on' has solved and always will solve the problems of the human race.*

Calvin Coolidge

The subconscious has a marvellous ability to solve problems. Have you ever gone to bed with a worry on your mind? You may have lain awake for hours trying to solve it. Next morning, or in the middle of the night, you find the answer. While you have been sleeping your subconscious mind has found the solution and your conscious mind tells you what it is.

Let's say you are taking an exam. The night before, just before going to sleep, say to yourself, 'I will pass that exam! I will not fail. I will pass, I will pass.' Put this into your subconscious mind (the best computer in the world).

If you tell yourself, 'I won't pass, I haven't prepared enough for it, I just know I won't pass,' then you won't pass ...

You can do anything you wish, it's completely up to you.

Most of us get bogged down with habits. We can't be bothered getting out of our own way. Some parents tell their children from birth, 'You are stupid, you are ugly, you won't make it.' They don't feel good about themselves and their children inherit their habits of low esteem. On the other hand, some parents are so successful they intimidate their children, destroying their self worth.

Please, don't have a chip on your shoulder! It's so unnecessary to feel unliked, ugly, poor, depressed, a slob, a dope.

Take people who run late for appointments; no matter what, they always run late. They will have five minutes to spare, decide to buy the paper and sure enough they still run late. Actually they have programmed their computer to run late and can't break the pattern.

Untidy and messy people: You'll find their appearance, their car, study, house are all messy. They'll make all kinds of excuses, they'll tell you they are too busy to be tidy. No, they are actually running around in circles getting nowhere. It's the *tidy and organised people* who have the tidy minds and get things done. (I concede that sometimes there appear to be exceptions to the rule!)

People who are always broke will always be broke; even if they were to win Lotto, within two years they'd be broke again. Then on the other hand, people who are rich and lose all their money on some venture will come up and be rich again. The rich get richer and the poor get poorer!

... IT'S ALL IN THE MIND!

Within each of us lies the power of our own consent to health and sickness; to riches and poverty; to freedom and slavery!
    It is we who control these and not another.

Richard Bach, *Illusions*

If a man says he can
If a man says he cannot
He is right either way ...

Break the patterns, the habits, the inherited genes. Programme your subconscious to change; make yourself into the *new you!*

It's All a State of Mind

If you think you are beaten, you are.
If you think you dare not, you won't.
If you like to win, but don't think you can,
It's almost a cinch you won't.
If you think you'll lose, you're lost.
For out in the world you'll find success begins with a fellow's will.
It's all in a state of mind.
For many a game is lost before even a play is run.
And many a coward fails before even his work has begun.

Think big and your deeds will grow.
Think small and you'll fall behind.
Think that you can and you will.

It's all in a state of mind.
If you think you're outclassed, you are.
You've got to think high to rise.
You've got to be sure of yourself before you can ever win a prize.
Life's battles don't always go to the stronger or faster man,
But sooner or later the man who wins is the fellow who thinks he can.

Anon.

Happiness Needs a Project

It is important to have a project. Have you noticed when you are in the middle of a project you are the happiest? Have you noticed when you are finished you look around for something else to give you interest? Someone once said to me, 'The day you get up in the morning and you have nothing to look forward to is a very unhappy day!'

Write down your goals. Number them, the small ones first, big ones last.

For example:
1. Learn the piano
2. Grow a herb garden
3. Be organised
4. Write a book
5. Learn French
6. Send the children to a private school
7. Buy a new car
8. Buy a boat
9. Take a trip around the world
10. Buy a better house

ALWAYS AIM HIGH
NEVER SETTLE FOR SECOND BEST

Think Big

If somebody thinks that when he or she makes a million dollars he or she will be happy, that person is a very great fool.

Leo Buscaglia

Material possessions don't make you happy, although they will make a change for a while. Remember you can have the best car and house in the world and one miserable marriage and be desperately unhappy. Take a look at the movie stars; most of them obtain wealth and material possessions and most of them seem to be unhappy. Happiness comes from within, the same as despair.

Enjoy life and make it happen for you. Positive thinkers dwell on what they want. Live each day as it comes, forget last year's problems—they have gone. Begin today ...

THIS IS THE FIRST DAY OF THE REST OF YOUR LIFE

Your Job or No Job?

If I were to do an interview to find out if someone was happy, my first question would be, 'Do you like your job?'

Most of us spend half our life at work, so we must feel satisfied and happy in what we are working at. Nobody can possibly be happy if they hate their job.

With all the unemployment today, it is certainly difficult to change jobs, but nothing is impossible. Every night when you go to bed, programme your subconscious mind; imagine yourself in a job you like, tell yourself you'll do your utmost to find something better and before you know it, you will.

To achieve happiness in your employment is to be needed, to feel your input is heading somewhere, to have an aim, a challenge to work for, to socialise and to be happy amongst your fellow workers. These things make the difference.

People who are dependent on social benefits, handouts, their parents' money and the like and who have nothing wrong with them—in other words the 'gunnas'—you may be sure, sooner or later, will lose their self worth and self drive. Their minds will become programmed to think negative and in the end they won't want to work as they are emotionally depressed. Don't let that butterfly elude you!

Relationships

My happiness is me not you
Not only because you may be temporary
But also because you want me to be what I am not.
I cannot be happy when I change
Merely to satisfy your selfishness.
Nor can I feel content when you criticise me for not thinking your thoughts.
Or for seeing like you do.
You call me a rebel.
And each time I have rejected your beliefs you have rebelled against
*   mine.*
I do not try to mould your mind.
I know you are trying hard enough to be just you.
And I cannot allow you to tell me what to be—
For I am concentrating on being me.

Anon.
Quoted in Leo Buscaglia's great book, *Living, Loving and Learning*

Woe be unto you if you give yourself totally to another! You're lost forever! Nobody can do it for you, they can give you encouragement, but it's up to you.

> *Give your hearts, but not into each other's keeping.*
> *For only the hand of life can contain your hearts.*
> *And stand together yet not too near together,*
> *For the pillars of the temple stand apart,*
> *And the oak tree and the cypress grow not in each other's shadow.*

Kahlil Gilbran, *The Prophet*

Your main responsibility is to yourself because if you don't belong to yourself, you can't give anything to anybody else. Be stimulating and not always predictable. This will help your relationship to work and to last.

This world and the people who live in it are becoming unhappier by the minute.

IT IS UP TO YOU TO CHANGE IT!

Today we are lucky if two adult people live in the same house. Talk about a lonely world! Our children are living with single parents. Our youth leave home at an early age. Our elderly are in nursing and retirement homes. One in every three people is divorced. A lot of the world is at war. People are dying of hunger. The seas, rivers and atmosphere are being destroyed by chemicals and pollution. The forests are being raped. Animals are becoming extinct.

Television is helping to destroy the family unit also. People watch on average five hours of television a day; this has an effect on our children. Instead of watching videos they should be outside playing, using their imagination and enjoying nature. The evening chats around the dining table at night have gone, replaced by TV trays on laps, each person sitting in their own lonely little world. How sad! Sure, television is a boom for the elderly and lonely and some programmes are informative and interesting, but not for five hours a day!

No wonder our world and the people in it are not very happy.

RIGHT: *Keeping in touch with friends is essential to your happiness*

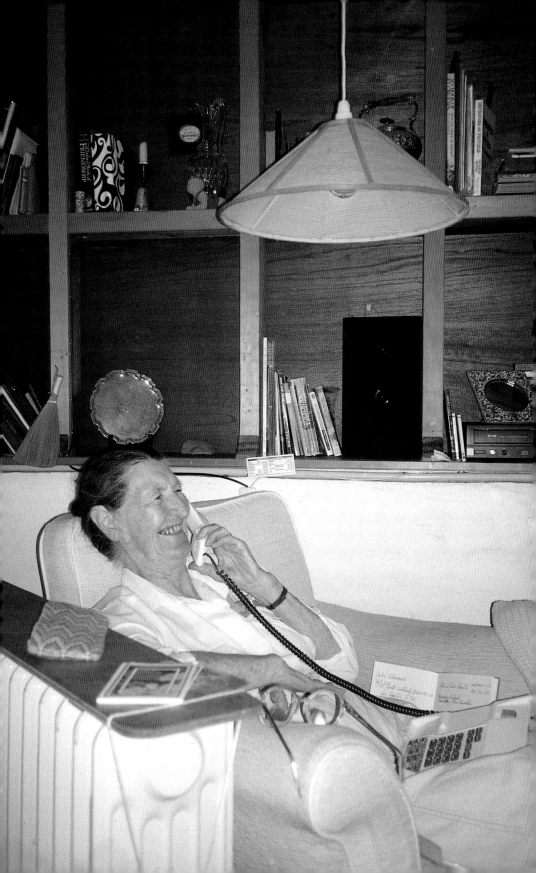

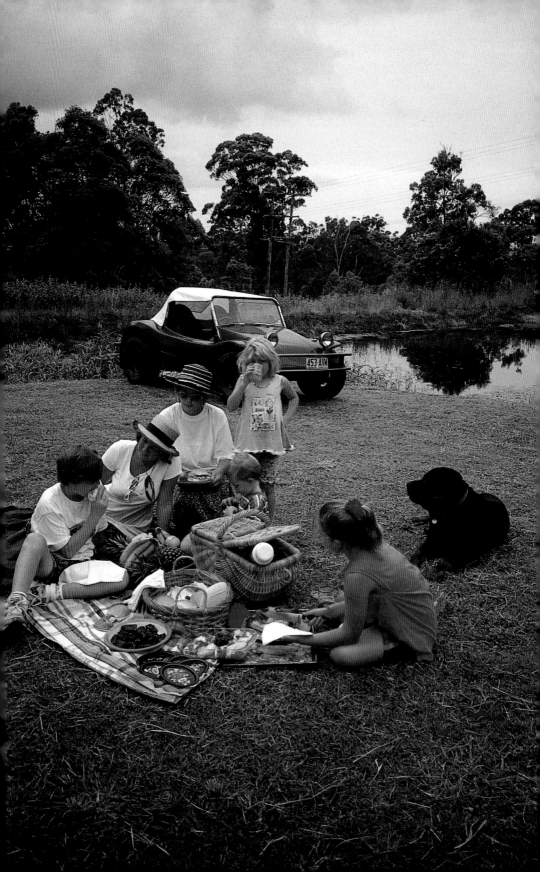

This poem says it all ...

Something's going wrong
With the singer and the song
And the music isn't gentle any more.
There's a mist across the moon
And the sun's too hot at noon
And the house is dark behind the broken door.

Where the flowers used to grow
Withered leaves are hanging low
And a constant shadow lies across the floor.
There's a strange and empty sky
Where the wild birds used to fly
And I never tasted bitter rain before.

Will the grass be gone from underneath the sky?
Will the golden flowers wither soon and die?
Will the fire burn up the land?
Will the sea fill up with sand?
Will the last word ever spoken be 'why'?

Someone's lost the plan for the brotherhood of man
And no-one's trying to find it any more.
The wind's become a sigh
For those who hate and those who die
And the waves are black and slow along the shore.

Anon.

For heaven's sake, don't you lose your plan for the brotherhood of man.

Today, go out and do something for someone. It need not be a big deal—a small surprise; a bouquet of flowers; a cheery letter or note; a small gift; a friendly word; a visit to a friend—but do something.

LEFT: *Relaxing by the dam with a picnic featuring salad rolls, Vine Leaf Parcels with Rich Mango Sauce (page 136) and Cabbage and Rice Rolls in Tomato Sauce (page 137)*

All your stress and anxiety will go. You will feel happy. The butterfly of happiness will come and softly sit on your shoulder.

Two men looked out from prison bars;
One saw mud, the other stars!

I'm sure you are going to see stars.

At the end of the day,
Just kneel and say:
'Thank you, Lord, for my work and play;
I've tried to be good,
For I know that I should.'
That's a prayer for the end of the day!
So when the new dawn begins to break,
Just lift up your eyes, let your heart awake;
Be ready to meet what the day may send,
And be ready to greet every man as a friend.
Nobody knows what a power you have found,
So do what you can for the others around;
Carry them high when they seem to be low,
As on your way you go.
At the end of the day.

Donald O'Keefe

CHAPTER 6 # Healthy Eating

Introduction to Recipes

As people who have read my books will know, it is my belief that of all the bad habits humans have invented, the practice of cooking is probably the most dangerous to our long-term health. To explain in detail why would take up the rest of this book, but perhaps it is sufficient here to say that the effect of heat on food is to destroy natural enzymes which would otherwise assist in its digestion, while at the same time, heat, according to its intensity and duration, alters the food's chemical structure, lessening its nutritional value. This of course places an increased load on the digestive system, which is then faced with the additional burden of getting rid of various toxic by-products which otherwise would not occur.

Whereas the human race would suffer few health problems if the practice of cooking was totally abandoned, there are many reasons why this would be completely impossible, one of them being that many products upon which people depend for sustenance, such as grains, have to be cooked to be digestible. Similarly, while animal foods can be digested raw, they must be cooked to make them palatable.

Apart from all this, cooking is so deeply ingrained in human culture and conveys so many taste advantages, that very few people, no matter how health conscious, are prepared to abandon it entirely.

Toni and I are no exceptions to the rule and have our little indulgences from time to time, but it is more difficult for her to be strict than it is for me, and there are two reasons for this. The first is that I am thirteen years older than she is and have watched many of my old contemporaries go down the drain—some completely. The second is that in the past she has always believed that to be a good wife it is essential to be a good cook, and because she has a compulsion to excel at anything she undertakes, I can state now with confidence that she is the best cook in the country.

Because all of the recipes in this book are low in fat, protein and salt, the

resultant dishes, whether cooked or not, even if eaten freely will avoid most of the blood impurities that lead to many common health problems such as blocked arteries, arthritis, diabetes and so on. To aim even higher for a guarantee against all problems, including cancer, remember that your choice should mainly be the raw fruits and salads which provide maximum health benefits.

Ross Horne

The first consideration in adopting a healthy diet is to stop eating foods which upsets the chemistry of the body and lead to disease. These foods are:

Fat or oil of any kind
Butter or margarine of any kind
Peanut butter
Cheese, milk, cream, yoghurt (unless non-fat)
Olives
Nuts
Eggs (egg whites are okay)
Any fried food
Sugar, raw sugar, brown sugar, molasses, treacle, syrup, etc
White bread, white rice or other processed cereals
Pies, cakes, pastries containing sugar, butter, shortening or salt
Biscuits, cookies, bread, cereals containing sugar, butter, shortening
Commercial cereals, cornflakes, etc
Soft drinks or other drinks containing sugar
Canned fruit or vegetables
Canned or packaged juices
James, jellies, sweets, chocolate, candy
Ice-cream
Tomato sauce, tartare sauce
Salt or any salted food (including monosodium glutamate)
Mustard, pickles, Worcestershire sauce, curry, mayonnaise
Sulphured dried fruits
Canned or packaged foods containing preservatives, sugar or salt

So what is there left to eat and drink? Quite a lot, if you think about it. Particularly fruit, vegetables, grains and legumes.

84

So here are the ALLOWED FOODS:

- All vegetables and fruit, preferably fresh. If cooked, steam them on a steaming rack for just a few minutes and remove as soon as they are softening. Salads of sliced beans, mushrooms, zucchinis, etc. can be made more interesting by adding fresh herbs and squeezed lemon or orange juice. Potatoes should be peeled, as they contain an alkaloid called solanine which, in high levels, is poisonous. Solanine levels are highest in stored potatoes which have turned green in colour. Avoid the excessive consumption of raw onion and garlic as they upset the taste buds and cause you to crave heavy foods.
- Legumes are allowed, except for soya beans which have too much fat. Brown lentils stewed with chopped tomatoes and onions, with herbs added instead of salt, are delicious.
- All fresh fruit is allowed but for people who have highly elevated triglyceride levels, fruit should be limited to four or five pieces a day at spaced intervals until triglycerides reduce. One piece of citrus fruit—orange, lemon, grapefruit, etc.—should be eaten each day.
- Wholegrain pita and rye bread.
- Wholegrain spaghetti and wholegrain macaroni.
- Wholegrain salt-free and fat-free crackers are available from health stores.
- Brown unpolished rice.

You may eat as much as you like of the allowed foods (except dried fruit) and still lose excess weight. It is better to eat frequent small snacks rather than large well-spaced meals. This avoids the high levels of blood sugar which follow large meals, and which result in an undesirable increase in blood fats.

At first the food may seem plain and uninteresting. This is because your taste buds are jaded by the exotic flavours of modern foods and spices, especially by the excessive use of salt and sugar. These tastes were acquired; after a short time, your palate will readjust and will appreciate the natural flavours of food.

Buying Food

Your main supplier of food will be the greengrocer. If you use a supermarket, most of your purchases will be fruit and vegetables, as nearly everything else they sell is processed and therefore undesirable. If you spend a little time reading the labels on packets and cans you will see why. If you have to use canned vegetables, never buy anything packed in oil, and select a brand free of sugar and salt. If this is not possible, avoid using the liquid from the can.

Bread must be 100% wholegrain and contain no shortening, sugar or salt. Many people bake their own. Unpolished rice, wholegrain products such as flour, spaghetti, macaroni, etc. are easily obtainable, if not from the supermarket, at all health food stores.

Raw oats, cracked wheat, dried beans, lentils, peas, etc can also be bought in these stores. An important thing to remember is that many health food store proprietors know very little about nutrition, and they enthusiastically sell loads of food filled with fat and sugar of some sort.

In some of the recipes wine is used to give flavour, but no harm comes of this because the alcohol contained in the wine evaporates away during cooking.

Useful Hints

- ❖ Always try to serve a raw mixed salad at either lunch or dinner.
- ❖ Start the meal with soup; you can make large quantities and store it in the freezer.
- ❖ Emphasise the vegetable content of a dish and minimise the meat or fish content, using it more as a flavouring. Spaghetti, pasta and rice dishes permit minimum quantities of meat.
- ❖ Try to balance the green and yellow vegetables with at least one or two starchy vegetables, such as potatoes, brown rice, etc. Steaming the vegetables retains their flavour and nourishment.
- ❖ Serve wholegrain bread; it is more satisfying to the appetite.
- ❖ Use generously fat-free, sugar-free and salt-free wholegrain crackers such as Ryvita, Rye Krisp and Scandinavian flat bread. Salt-free Mexican chips and vegetable chips are obtainable at health food stores.
- ❖ Avoid vinegar as it retards the digestion of starches.

- Use plenty of lemon to flavour salads and vegetables. Garlic and herbs can be used.
- Non-stick cookwear allows cooking without fat and without greasing the pans. Avoid using pressure cookers, microwave ovens or aluminium utensils. The higher the temperature in cooking, the more the nutritional value of the food is depleted. Aluminium enters the food and is toxic to the body. It is preferable to use stainless steel, enamel or ceramic utensils. Pyrex or Corningware are good. For sauteing without oil, use a Silverstone pan or baking dish.
- If meat of any kind is used, cook it well first and chill to congeal the fat so it can be removed. The meat can be reheated.
- In recipes calling for eggs, use the whites only, as the yolks are high in cholesterol and fat. Mix with skim milk to make up the volume, or use double the amount of egg white.
- To sweeten dishes, use grated apple or mashed banana or other fruit.
- The cheese used in some of the recipes is special non-fat or very low fat cottage or ricotta cheese.
- Steaming is better than boiling because more nutrients are retained. Cook as briefly as possible, because high temperatures and overcooking severely reduce the nutritional quality of the food. The most harmful foods are those deep-fried in oil.
- For quick steaming, cut vegetables into small pieces. Root vegetables, which take longer, should be cut into smaller pieces than other vegetables. Steam vegetables only sufficiently to render them chewable.
- After juicing a lemon, wrap and freeze the skin, so that if a recipe calls for lemon rind you don't have to waste a fresh lemon.
- Bananas will not darken when peeled if they are coated with lemon juice.
- Freeze bananas that are about to over-ripen; make into ice blocks or blend into smoothies.
- Parsley can be preserved in the freezer—chop and place in plastic bag, freeze and use as required.
- Parsley and herbs are most easily chopped fine in a Mouli hand-operated chopper.
- Garlic can be preserved in the freezer. To use, peel and chop cloves before thawing.
- Vegetables are best kept in the refrigerator in airtight plastic bags or containers.

❖ To dry a large quantity of wet salad greens quickly, keeping them crisp, place in a pillow case and spin dry in the washing machine for a few minutes. To keep them crisp until serving, cover with wet kitchen paper and put in refrigerator.

❖ To remove the core from a lettuce, hit the core end once sharply against the countertop. The core will then twist out. This method avoids the brown marks caused by cutting.

❖ To store peeled potatoes, cover in cold water and add a few drops of vinegar. In the refrigerator they will last up to four days.

❖ To peel tomatoes, soak in boiling water for a few moments; the skin then comes off easily.

❖ Fruit and vegetables should be thoroughly washed to remove traces of chemical insecticides.

❖ Home grown or organically grown fruits and vegetables are considered superior because they have not been sprayed (unless you sprayed them yourself) with chemical insecticides, and have not spent extended periods in cold storage.

❖ Juicers which extract juice by grinding and pressure action are superior to the centrifugal type. Juices should be prepared just before drinking. Vegetable juices are good, but fruit is better eaten whole to gain the best assimilation of the natural fruit sugars.

❖ Canned, packaged or processed foods should be avoided. Apart from whatever additives they may contain, they are completely devoid of natural enzymes. If such foods must be used, read the labels carefully to avoid salt, sugar and fat. If canned food is packed in salt water or oil, pour all liquids off before using. Processed meats are the most harmful foods. They can also cause allergies.

DO NOT CHEAT!
DO NOT CHEAT!
DO NOT CHEAT!

Salt Substitures

Saltless surprise: 2 teaspoons garlic powder and 1 teaspoon each of basil and oregano. Mix ingredients in a blender. (Add rice afterwards to prevent the mixture caking.)

Pungent salt substitute: 3 teaspoons basil, 2 teaspoons each of savory, celery seed, ground cumin, sage and marjoram, and 1 teaspoon lemon thyme. Mix well then powder with a mortar and pestle.

Spicy saltless seasoning: 1 teaspoon each of cloves, pepper and coriander seed (crushed), 2 teaspoons paprika, and 1 tablespoon rosemary. Mix ingredients in a blender.

Recipes from *The FDA Consumer*, the journal of the US Food and Drug Administration

Eating Out

It is almost impossible to obtain suitable food in an ordinary restaurant. Even health food restaurants use lashings of oil on salads and in cooking. The best thing to do if you are intent on maintaining your diet is to explain to the waiter you are a vegetarian and that you are not allowed any fat or oil and ask, say, for soup followed by plain vegetables or salad. Waiters are usually very cooperative and do their best, even though the food you eventually receive is usually very salty. A smorgasbord restaurant is okay because you can serve yourself all the salad and vegetables you want. Use lemon juice on the salad.

The food in many Chinese restaurants is very high in fat, cholesterol and salt. However, you can always get steamed vegetables and boiled rice which make a satisfying meal.

Social Drinking

Avoiding alcohol is pretty simple—you can just ask for something non-alcoholic with soda water or even a small white wine or beer mixed with soda water. This allows you to enjoy convivial company and often you will find others copying your technique.

Part of the enjoyment of beer drinking is the visual effect of colour, a frothy head, and condensation on the glass. The sensation of taste derives largely from the correct temperature of the beer and the tingling sensation of the carbon dioxide bubbles. By pouring a small quantity of stout into a beer glass and then topping it up with cold soda water you have a refreshing drink which looks like beer, has a head, tastes like beer, and yet is 80% soda water ... Cheers!

Conversion Tables

Weights and Measures

Converting solid measures

Metric	Imperial	
30 g	1 oz	(actual weight 28.5 g)
125 g	4 oz	(actual weight 114 g)
250 g	8 oz	(actual weight 227 g)
375 g	12 oz	(actual weight 341 g)
500 g	1 lb	(actual weight 454 g)
1 kg	2 lb	(actual weight 908 g)

Converting liquid measures

Metric	Imperial
30 ml	1 fl oz
60 ml (¼ metric cup)	2 fl oz
125 ml (½ metric cup)	4 fl oz
150 ml (¼ pint)	5 fl oz
250 ml	8 fl oz
300 ml	10 fl oz
600 ml	20 fl oz

Cup measures

	Metric	Imperial
1 cup sugar	250 g	8 oz
1 cup flour	155 g	5 oz
1 cup shortening (butter, margarine, etc.)	250 g	8 oz
1 cup honey, golden syrup, etc.	375 g	12 oz
1 cup fresh breadcrumbs	60 g	2 oz
1 cup mixed fruit	185 g	6 oz
1 cup nuts, chopped	125 g	4 oz
1 cup rice, uncooked	220 g	7 oz

Oven temperatures

Electric temperatures	°Celsius	°Fahrenheit
Very slow	120	250
Slow	150	300
Moderately slow	160–180	325–350
Moderate	190–200	375–400
Moderately hot	220–230	425–450
Hot	250–260	475–500

Gas temperatures	°Celsius	°Fahrenheit
Very slow	120	250
Slow	140–150	275–300
Moderately slow	160	325
Moderate	180	350
Moderately hot	190	375
Hot	200–230	400–450

Daily Eating Programme

Breakfast

A glass of carrot and celery juice a day is said to melt the fat away. Drink a glass of juice before or with breakfast.

Caffeine stimulates the nervous system and upsets the blood sugar. Instead of tea or coffee, drink a cup of herbal tea.

Allow your digestive system to have a comparative rest from the previous night to the following lunchtime.

For breakfast always the same:

Fruit salad or fresh fruit, enough to satisfy your hunger. Eat bananas when you feel particularly hungry. If you are still hungry throughout the morning, eat a banana or apple, melon or a bunch of grapes. Melons are full of water so eat them before other fruits.

Try a fruit smoothie!

½ cup fresh orange juice combined with ½ cup apple juice or 1 cup skim milk. To liquid add 1 frozen or fresh banana, an apple or ½ paw paw (papaya) and ½ avocado, or 1 cup of any fruit you desire.

Place juice or milk with banana and fruit of choice in blender and liquefy. Makes 1 glass.

Lunch

Fresh juice
Pita bread filled with salad
Wholemeal bread sandwiches
Ryvita biscuits with filling
Herb damper with filling
Soups
Salads
Baked potato with filling
Baked sweet potato or pumpkin
Pasta
Rice

When working away from home it is so easy to pick up fatty junk food from takeaway outlets. Don't fall for it! Instead buy healthy salads, fruit salads, filled pita bread, salad sandwiches. Why not take a home-made sandwich and fruit from home? The main thing is to develop *good* eating habits.

Dinner

Fresh vegetable juice
Salad
Soup
Rice
Pasta
Chicken
Fish

Serve main dishes with a salad of your choice, steamed vegetables or rice. A salad followed by a thick hearty soup is very satisfying. Try to avoid eating a lot of animal protein at meals. Cooking destroys the natural enzymes in food, so eat as much raw food as possible. If you are still hungry after your main meal, eat some fruit.

Juices

All juices should be made from fresh vegetables and fruit and should be consumed within fifteen minutes of preparation, before they begin to oxidise and lose their vitamin and enzyme content. Canned, cartoned and bottled juices are totally undesirable, and are absolutely forbidden by advocates of healthy eating. Whether or not they contain preservatives, they are completely devoid of natural enzymes.

Vegetable juices are preferred to fruit juices as fruit juice is too concentrated in sugar, even though it is natural sugar. It is better to eat fruit whole, thoroughly chewing it, for best nourishment. Fruit juice is acceptable if the fruit cannot be chewed but it should be taken in small quantities at spaced intervals to avoid big increases in blood sugar. Fruit juice is also acceptable as a sweetener mixed with vegetable juices. Juice made from raisins blended with water also adds sweetness to other juices.

Juices are best extracted by a pressure type juicing machine as high speed centrifugal type juicers are thought to reduce the quality of juice by way of oxidation. Juice can be extracted from vegetables and fruit by first pulping the flesh in a blender, then squeezing the pulp in a

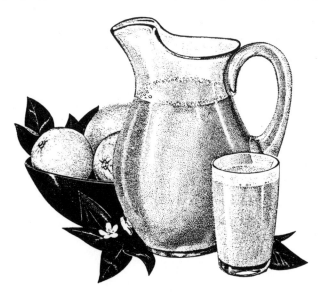

cheesecloth bag. The pressure type juice extractors are manually or electrically powered and work something like a meat grinder, first grinding the vegetable matter, then forcing it through a tapered spout so that the juice is squeezed out. This type of juicer was developed to extract the juice of wheatgrass.

Wheatgrass juice, although considered to be the most nutritious of juices, is not palatable at first taste. It is used mainly to provide concentrated nourishment to invalids and should be taken in very small quantities (30-60 ml) diluted with water.

Vegetable juices are the builders and regenerators of the body. They contain all the amino acids, minerals, salts, enzymes and vitamins needed by the human body, provided that they are used fresh, raw, and without preservatives, and that they have been properly extracted from the vegetables.

Green juices (containing chlorophyll) may be made from alfalfa, bean sprouts, broccoli, buckwheat, cabbage, celery, Chinese celery, chives, cucumbers, fennel, green beans, green peppers, lettuce, parsley, shallots, spinach, turnips, wheatgrass, watercress.

Fruit juices (which contain sugars) may be made from apples, apricots, avocados, bananas, blackberries, cherries, grapefruits, grapes, guavas, honeydew melon, cumquats, lemons, limes, mangoes, nectarines, oranges, papapas, peaches, pears, persimmons, pineapples, plums, pomegranates, raspberries, rock melon, tangerines, watermelon.

Different juices combine well to provide flavour and nourishment.

Juice combinations

Avocado and:	lemon
Apple and:	carrot
	banana
	celery
Banana and:	mint
	papaya (pawpaw)
Brussel sprouts and:	string beans
	broccoli
Carrot and:	apple
	celery
	lettuce
	spinach
	turnip

	watercress
	fennel
	orange
	string beans
	cucumber
Cabbage and:	celery
	parsley
	apple
Celery and:	cucumber
	carrot
	parsley
	turnip
	spinach
	lettuce
	string beans
	cucumber
Cucumber and:	apple
Pineapple and:	fresh coconut
Tomato and:	alfalfa
	carrot
	watercress
	lettuce
	avocado
	celery
	green pepper

Wheatgrass

Dr Ann Wigmore of Boston many years ago restored her own health by adopting a diet based on raw grasses, which she later demonstrated contains all the nutrients to sustain a human in perfect health. A great number of tests carried out by Dr Wigmore showed that wheatgrass juice was the most nourishing of all juices. She has since demonstrated the effectiveness of a raw fruit and vegetable diet, supplemented by generous quantities of wheatgrass juice, in nourishing and cleansing the bodies of many patients with advanced cancer, restoring them to sound health again. Whereas wheat and wheat products are difficult to digest and provoke allergic responses in many people, wheatgrass is much more nourishing and has not been known to produce adverse reactions. Juicing the wheatgrass permits taking in more of its con-centrated nourishment and this is considered important by Dr Wigmore for people whose bodies require all the nourishment they can get.

How to grow wheatgrass

Buy the wheat grain, preferably organically grown, from a health food store. Get a large tray such as a cake shop baking tray, or anything similar. Get some good soil, mix with wet peat moss if obtainable to provide good ventilation and drainage. Spread the soil 2.5 cm thick in the tray, leaving it loose and smooth on top, and form a trench along both sides.

Soak the seed 8 to 15 hours and allow to drain, preferably about 8 hours before planting.

Wet the soil without converting it to mud or leaving any puddles.

Spread a layer of seed so that all the surface of the soil is covered but no seeds are on top of one another. Cover the seed with wet news-paper. In warm, humid weather use four sheets and up to eight sheets in cold, dry weather. Cover the lot with a sheet of plastic but do not enclose so as to prevent air circulation.

On the fourth day remove the plastic and paper. Water the sprouts and place tray in the sunlight. Water every morning and in dry condi-tions keep the crop moist by more frequent light spraying. In a week the grass will be about seven inches tall and ready for harvesting.

Cut the greens close to the base to ensure getting all the best nutri-tional substances. The greens can be used as such, or juiced.

To ensure a continuous supply, several trays can be used, each with a crop at a different stage. After the crop is cut the mat of earth should be taken out and fresh earth substituted.

If the weather is severe and cold, wheatgrass can be grown indoors, although without sunlight the grass will not manufacture chlorophyll unless daylight-emitting fluorescent lights are used.

RIGHT: *Water, sunshine, a happy child ... a wonderful way to reduce stress*

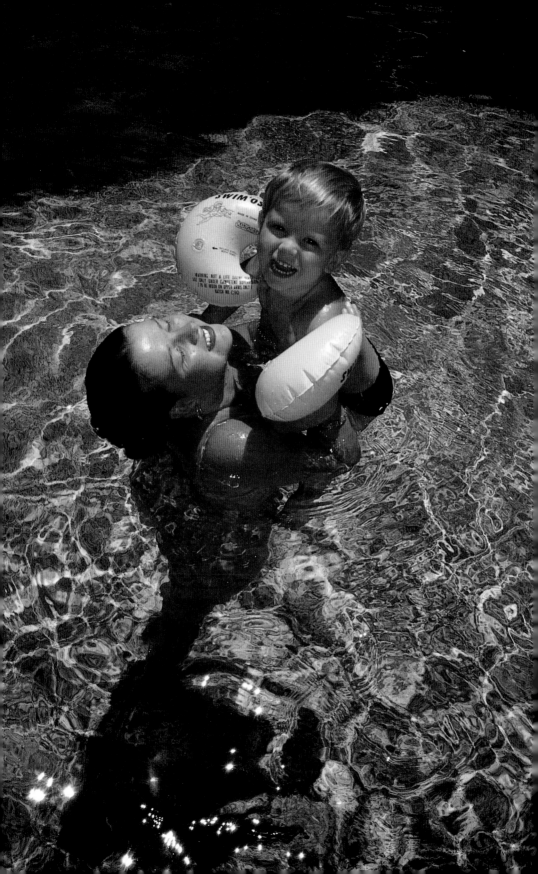

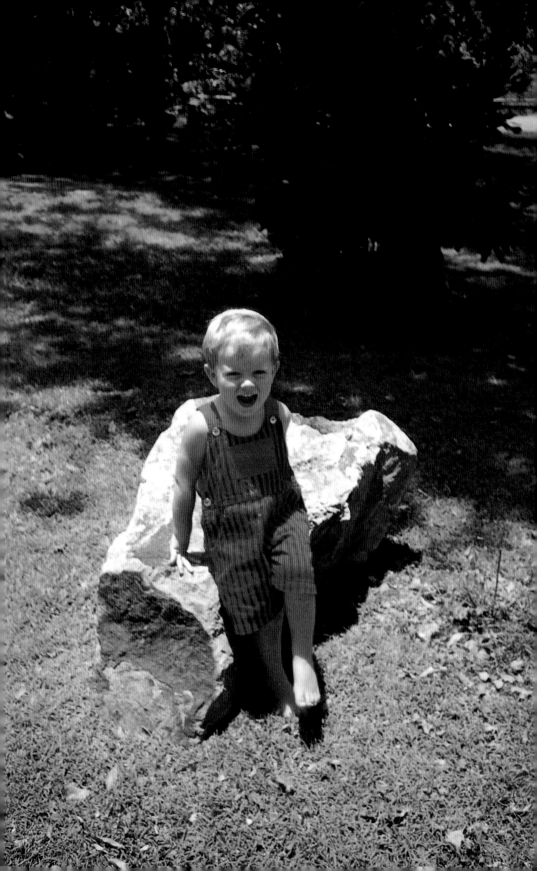

CHAPTER 7 Recipes

Soups

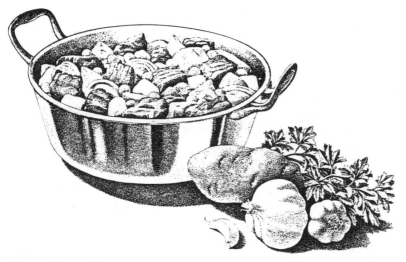

Hints from the range

❖ If fresh stock is to be used immediately, skim off as much surface fat as possible, then float an ice cube to congeal the rest. A piece of chilled lettuce will collect the remaining fat.

❖ Stocks may be frozen in ice cube trays; store the frozen cubes in plastic bags and use as needed.

❖ Stocks will last about five days in the refrigerator.

❖ Soups may be made into a main meal and served with a fresh garden salad. They are nourishing as well as slimming.

Chicken Stock

LEFT: Enjoy your children's happiness

8 cups water
1 boiling fowl (or chicken)
1 large white onion stuck with 3 cloves
2 tabs chopped celery
1 garlic clove
3 stalks celery and leaves
1 parsnip
2 carrots
pinch thyme
1 teas kelp
½ bay leaf
black pepper

Remove all skin and fat from fowl, cover with cold water and bring to boil. Reduce heat and simmer for 30 minutes. Drain off liquid, put into freezer until fat forms on top of stock, skim off floating particles and put through a strainer. Prepare vegetables, cut into slices and add to strained liquid and fowl. Simmer for one hour or until fowl is tender. Strain. Cool and keep in refrigerator. Stock may be frozen for future use. Cooking time 1½ to 2 hours.

Vegetable Stock

8 cups water
1 turnip
3 stalks celery
2 carrots
1 parsnip
1 onion stuck with 3 cloves
1 large tomato
3 garlic cloves (peeled)
½ bay leaf
pinch thyme
1 teas kelp
black pepper

Prepare vegetables and cut into thin slices. Bring to boil, cover and simmer for 30 minutes. Cool. Put through electric blender. Refrigerate or freeze.

Easy Stock

To 2 cups water add ingredients desired—garlic, onion, celery, fresh ginger, curry powder, tomato paste or various herbs of choice. Simmer for 20 minutes.

Fish Stock

8 cups water
4 fish heads plus bones and skin
1 celery stalk, chopped
2 onions, chopped
2 cloves garlic, crushed
1 tabs fresh ginger, chopped
1 bunch coriander roots
2 tabs coriander leaves, chopped
½ cup white wine

Prepare vegetables, add to water with herbs and fish heads, bones and skin. Bring to boil, cover and simmer for 30 minutes. Remove all bones. Puree in a blender and add white wine.

Slimmer's Vegetable Soup

6 cups chicken stock
2 onions, chopped
2 garlic cloves, crushed
2 parsnips, peeled and chopped
2 carrots, peeled and chopped
½ cup green beans, peeled and sliced
1 cup soaked barley
black pepper

Cook barley in water until soft, add to the stock and remaining ingredients. Simmer for 30 minutes. If a thick consistency is required, thicken with flour mixed with a little water. Serves 4.

Coconut Cream Soup with Prawns

1 cup fish stock
1 cup skim milk
200 ml coconut cream
4 shallots, chopped
½ cup white wine
20 green prawns (peeled and chopped)
1 tabs coriander, chopped
black pepper

In a saucepan add fish stock, milk, coconut cream, shallots, wine and prawns. Heat gently without boiling until prawns are red and tender. Serve with coriander and pepper. Serves 4.

Carrot and Orange Soup

4 cups chicken stock
4 large carrots, peeled and cut into slices
2 leeks (white part), cleaned, peeled and thinly sliced
2 teas honey
1 teas ground ginger
1 teas dried mustard powder
1 teas cornflour mixed with a little water
juice and rind of 1 orange
2 tabs mint
1 teas nutmeg
cornflour

To stock add carrots, leeks, honey, ginger and mustard. Bring to boil, simmer until carrots are tender (about 30 minutes) then thicken with cornflour. Stir in orange juice and rind, blend until smooth. Reheat without boiling and serve garnished with mint and nutmeg. Serves 4.

Winter Soup à la Montville

4 cups chicken stock
2 parsnips, peeled and chopped
2 small potatoes, peeled and diced
1 cup pumpkin, peeled and chopped
2 carrots, peeled and chopped

1 tomato, peeled and chopped
2 tabs coriander
1 teas cumin
1 teas nutmeg
½ cup ground pine nuts
¼ cup parsley and basil, chopped
4 slices bread
4 tabs natural yoghurt
black pepper

To chicken stock add all ingredients except the last five. Simmer soup for 20 minutes or until vegetables are tender. Brush bread sparingly with a little low-fat oil. Sprinkle pine nuts, parsley and basil on top of bread slices, bake on an oven tray for 20 minutes. Cut into croutons, skim a tablespoon of yoghurt around each soup bowl, add croutons and sprinkle with black pepper. Serves 4.

Creamy Scallop Chowder

2 medium potatoes, diced
1 small carrot, chopped
1 stalk celery, chopped
4 shallots, chopped
3 cups fish stock
½ bay leaf
½ teas fresh thyme
½ teas turmeric
freshly ground pepper
500 g (1 lb) scallops
½ cup dry white wine
1 cup blended ricotta cheese

Place potatoes, carrot, celery and shallots in a large pot, cover with fish stock and bring to boil. Add bay leaf, thyme, turmeric and pepper. Simmer, covered, until vegetables are tender. Remove bay leaf and transfer mixture to blender. Blend until smooth. Meanwhile saute scallops in wine for about 5 minutes. Stir in ricotta cheese and combine the mixture with the pureed vegetable broth. Heat through, garnish with paprika, parsley and pepper. Serves 4.

Soup à l'Oignon

4 cups chicken stock
½ cup dry white wine
4 large onions, thinly sliced
2 garlic cloves, crushed
1 tabs plain flour
2 teas soy sauce (low salt)
black pepper

Topping
4 slices French bread
1 cup grated low-fat Swiss cheese
¼ cup freshly grated parmesan cheese

Slowly brown the onions and garlic in a non-stick frypan with a little water. Cook until the onions turn dark brown (about 15 minutes). Stir with a wooden spoon to scrape the brown off the bottom of the pan. Add flour and cook for about 2 minutes. Add wine and cook a further 2 minutes. In a saucepan combine onions with stock, soy sauce and pepper and simmer for 1 hour. Transfer soup to heatproof individual bowls. Top each bowl with a slice of bread covered with Swiss cheese and sprinkled with parmesan. Bake covered for 15 minutes at 180°C (325°F), then uncover and bake a further 10 minutes. Serves 4.

Creamy Potato and Herb Soup

3 cups chicken stock
4 medium potatoes, peeled and chopped
2 leeks (white part), cleaned, peeled and thinly sliced
1 tabs fresh coriander
1 tabs fresh chives
1 tabs fresh oregano
1 teas nutmeg
1 cup skim milk
1 tabs parsley
black pepper

To stock add potatoes, leeks and herbs, bring to boil and reduce heat. Simmer until potatoes are tender. Blend mixture with milk until smooth, garnish with parsley and pepper. Serves 4.

Fennel, Lime and Ginger Soup

3 cups chicken stock
2 medium fennel bulbs, chopped
1 onion, chopped
1 clove garlic, crushed
1 apple, peeled and chopped
2 celery stalks, chopped
1 teas ginger, chopped
juice of 1 lime
½ cup skim milk

Add fennel, onion, garlic, apple, celery and ginger to stock. Bring to boil, reduce heat and simmer for about 20 minutes, add lime juice and milk. Garnish with fennel leaves and a slice of lime. Serves 4.

Two-tone Green and White Soup

½ bunch broccoli
½ cauliflower
1 medium onion, chopped
2 cloves garlic, chopped
1 large potato, chopped
2 stalks celery, chopped
2 tabs fresh coriander
3 cups chicken stock
1 cup skim milk
dash black pepper
mock sour cream (page 112)
red caviar

Chop broccoli and cauliflower into flowerets. Combine onion, garlic, potato, celery and 1 cup chicken stock in a saucepan and cook for 10 minutes until tender; meanwhile, cook the cauliflower in milk until tender then add to half the stock mixture. Blend until smooth in a blender. Steam broccoli until tender, mix with the remaining stock, blend and reheat. Ladle cauliflower soup into bowls with a spoon, then ladle broccoli mixture gently on top of the cauliflower. Make sure both soups are the same texture. Garnish each bowl with a dollop of mock sour cream and 1 teas red caviar. Serves 4.

Minty Green Soup

3 cups chicken stock
2 cloves garlic, crushed
1 cup spinach, washed and chopped
1 tabs cornflour blended with a little water
1 teas marjoram
1 teas soy sauce (low salt)
2 tabs mint finely chopped
2 mushrooms
lemon

Steam spinach until tender, drain well. Blend stock with herbs and spices. Add cornflour mixture and simmer for 10 minutes. Garnish with finely sliced mushrooms and lemon wedges.Serves 4.

Corn Chowder

4 cups chicken stock
1 onion, sliced
1 small bay leaf
2 tabs parsley, chopped
pinch of dried sage
freshly ground black pepper
1 cup potatoes, peeled and diced
3 teas plain flour
2½ cups corn kernels
1 cup skim milk
fresh coriander, chopped

To stock add onion slices, bay leaf, parsley, sage, pepper and potatoes. Cook until potatoes are tender. Thicken mixture with flour mixed with a little water. Add corn kernels and milk to the potato mixture and remove the bay leaf. Heat the chowder to a serving temperature. Garnish with coriander. Serves 4.

Orange-red Marbled Soup

4 cups chicken stock
1 cup skim milk
1 large potato, peeled and chopped

1 onion, chopped
1 teas ground cumin
1 teas ground coriander
1 large red pepper, seeded and finely chopped
1 butternut pumpkin
2 tabs chopped parsley
freshly ground pepper

To stock and milk add potato, onion, cumin, coriander. Cook until potato is tender. Halve the mixture and set aside. Meanwhile bake the pumpkin in the oven for about 30 minutes, peel when cooked, add to half the soup mixture and blend. Add the chopped red pepper to the other half of soup mixture, cook about 5 minutes until tender then blend. Pour pumpkin soup into a bowl, spoon red pepper mixture gently over. Garnish with chopped parsley and black pepper. Serves 4.

Garlic Potato Soup with Coriander

3 cups chicken stock
4 large potatoes, peeled and diced
2 cloves garlic, crushed
2 tabs fresh coriander, chopped
½ teas dry mustard
1 bay leaf
1 teas soy sauce (low salt)
1 cup mock sour cream (or skim milk)
nutmeg

To stock add potatoes, garlic, coriander, mustard, bay leaf and soy sauce. Bring to boil, simmer for about 20 minutes until tender. Remove bay leaf, add mock sour cream and blend until smooth. Garnish with a sprig of coriander and sprinkle with nutmeg. Serves 4.

Apple and Sultana Soup

4 apples
1 cup water
1 cup red wine
2 slices bread, crumbed
rind of 1 lemon

105

½ cup sultanas
2 tabs honey
2 teas brandy
¼ cup mock sour cream
1 teas cinnamon

Add apples to wine, water, bread and lemon rind, simmer until apples
are tender. Puree in a blender. Heat sultanas and honey in a saucepan,
bring to boil, stirring to prevent sticking. Simmer for 5 minutes, then
add brandy and mix with apple mixture. Garnish with sour cream and
sprinkle with cinnamon. Serves 4.

Cold Guacamole Soup

2 cups chicken stock
1 large ripe avocado
2 tabs fresh lemon juice
1 teas soy sauce (low salt)
dash cayenne pepper
1 cup mock sour cream (page 112)

Garnishes
mock sour cream
snipped chives
toasted almonds

Peel avocado and remove seed. Cut into small pieces and place in
blender. Add chicken stock and lemon juice, blend until smooth. Add
mock sour cream, soy sauce and pepper. Mix well and chill for 2 hours.
Toast almonds on a tray under grill until golden (about 5 minutes).
Pour soup into 4 individual bowls, garnish with an extra dollop of mock
sour cream, chives and almonds. Serves 4.

Gazpacho

2 large juicy tomatoes, peeled and seeded
½ green pepper, seeded and chopped
1 cucumber, peeled and chopped
½ cup chopped celery
1 small onion, chopped

2 cups tomato juice
1 avocado, seeded and chopped
1 teas soy sauce (low salt)
freshly ground black pepper

Garnishes
mock sour cream (page 112)
croutons

All vegetables must be very finely chopped. Combine all ingredients in a large bowl and chill overnight. Serve soup cold with a dollop of sour cream on top of each serving. Pass croutons in a bowl. Serves 4.

Fennel Soup with Pine Nuts

4 fennel bulbs cut into small pieces
1 onion, sliced
1 apple, chopped
4 cups chicken stock
¼ cup pine nuts
1 cup skim milk
juice 1 lemon
1 teas cinnamon

Simmer fennel, onion, apple in stock for 30 minutes until tender. Puree and reheat. Stir in pine nuts, milk, lemon juice. Top with cinnamon. Serves 4.

Smoked Salmon and Asparagus Chowder

1 cup chicken stock
1 cup skim milk
1 shallot, peeled and chopped
1 tabs plain flour
1 potato, peeled and diced
1 teas ground tarragon
1 cup asparagus, diced
2 smoked salmon fillets
freshly ground pepper

Add milk and shallots to stock, then mix in flour blended with a little water to thicken. Add potato and tarragon, cover and simmer until potato is tender (about 15 minutes). Meanwhile, in a separate saucepan steam asparagus until tender. Drain and set aside. Peel skin from salmon, cut flesh into bite sized pieces, add asparagus and salmon to potato mixture and heat. Season with pepper. Serves 4.

American Clam Chowder

500 g (1 lb) clams or pipis
1 large white fish fillet
3 cups fish stock
3 shallots, chopped
1 large potato, peeled and cubed
½ cup white wine
½ cup skim milk
1 teas turmeric
black pepper

Soak clams in water for 5 minutes, scrub and place in a saucepan of boiling water until clams open. Take out the ones that open first to prevent overcooking. Drain and remove liquid. Remove clams from shells. To the fish stock add shallots, potato, turmeric and bring to boil. Cook for 15 minutes or until potatoes are tender. Add skim milk, wine and clams. Reheat and season with pepper. Serves 4.

Toni's Minestrone

500 g (1 lb) shin of beef
1 veal knuckle
8 cups water
dash pepper
2 onions
2 garlic cloves
1 carrot, diced
1 stalk celery, chopped
3 large peeled tomatoes
2 level tabs tomato paste (unsalted)

1 can red kidney beans
1 cup fresh beans, chopped
2 cups spaghetti, broken into pieces
2 cups shredded cabbage

Put meats into a boiler, add water and pepper. Cover and simmer 1½ hours. Remove scum from stock and sides of pan. Add chopped onion, crushed garlic, carrot, celery, tomatoes, tomato paste. Simmer gently 30 minutes. Add can of kidney beans (including liquid) and fresh beans. Bring to boil, add spaghetti, cook until spaghetti is tender (about 20 minutes), adding cabbage during last 10 minutes. Remove meat, chop roughly and return to pot. Serve with a basket of warm crusty garlic bread. Serves 8.

The meat can be omitted, adding vegetable stock instead.

To make a stew, use less water, and thicken with plain wholewheat flour or cornflour.

Borsch

4 cups stock
1 large onion, sliced
2 cloves garlic, crushed
2 beetroot, peeled and cut into thin strips
1 carrot, peeled and cut into thin strips
1 stalk celery, chopped
1 large potato, diced
1 cup cooked haricot beans (or canned)
2 cups shredded cabbage
1 cup tomato juice
1 clove
juice ½ lemon
½ teas allspice
mock sour cream (page 112)
dill

To stock add onion, garlic, beetroot and carrot. Simmer gently until beetroot and carrot are almost done, then add potato, beans, cabbage, tomato juice and spices and cook till potato is tender. Add lemon juice. Serve topped with mock sour cream and dill. Serves 6.

Hungarian Soup

4 cups stock
4 small onions
2 garlic cloves
3 large ripe tomatoes, peeled and quartered
1 cup red cabbage, shredded
1 large cooking apple, finely chopped
½ teas allspice
2 teas paprika
coriander

Slice onions thinly and push into rings, add to stock with garlic, spices, tomatoes, red cabbage and apple. Cover and bring to boil. Simmer for 30 minutes. Serve with chopped coriander. Serves 6.

Dressings and Sauces

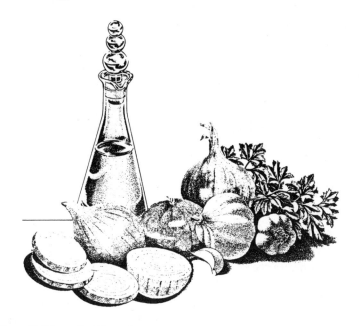

No-oil French Dressing

juice of 1 lemon
¼ cup cider vinegar
2 cloves garlic, crushed
¼ teas dill

½ cup water
¼ cucumber, finely chopped
¼ teas ground black pepper
2 teas chopped parsley

Mix ingredients in a blender and refrigerate overnight.

No-oil Italian Dressing

1 cup unsweetened apple juice
¼ cup lemon juice
½ teas oregano
1/8 teas thyme
½ cup cider vinegar
2 cloves garlic, crushed
½ teas paprika

Mix ingredients in blender and refrigerate overnight. The flavour
improves if left a day or two.

Coconut Dressing

½ cup coconut cream
½ cup coconut milk
1 teas grated lime rind
1 clove garlic, crushed
2 tabs lime juice
½ teas ground ginger

Blend together ground ginger with lime juice, blend in other ingredients. Add a little more ginger if desired. Chill. Serve with salad or fish.

Mock Sour Cream

½ cup skim milk
1 teas powdered skim milk
1 tabs cider vinegar or lemon juice
250 g (8 oz) ricotta cheese

Blend skim milk with powdered milk. Pour about ¼ cup of the milk into blender, add a small portion of the cheese. Blend and continue adding milk and cheese until the mixture has the consistency of sour cream. Add the lemon or vinegar. If a sourer taste is desired, add more lemon juice or vinegar. Mock sour cream keeps well for several days in an airtight container. Can be used as a topping for soups, blended into casseroles, or as topping for potatoes.

Avocado and Green Pepper Dressing

1 large avocado, peeled and stone removed
1 tabs canned green peppercorns, drained and crushed
1 tabs orange juice
1 teas grated orange rind
½ cup mock sour cream (see above)

Puree ingredients in a blender.

RIGHT: *A fireside meal of Quick Herbed Damper (page 158), Fish Pie on the left (page 153) and hearty Winter Soup à la Montville (page 100)*

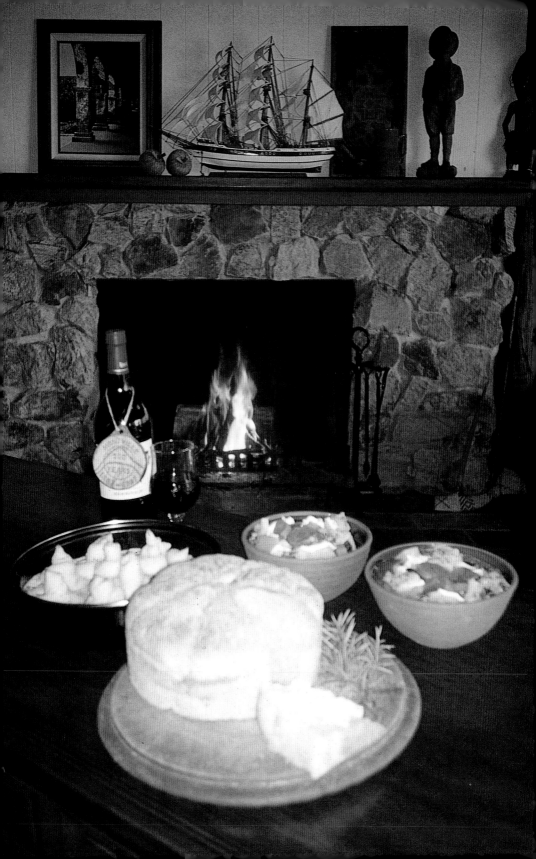

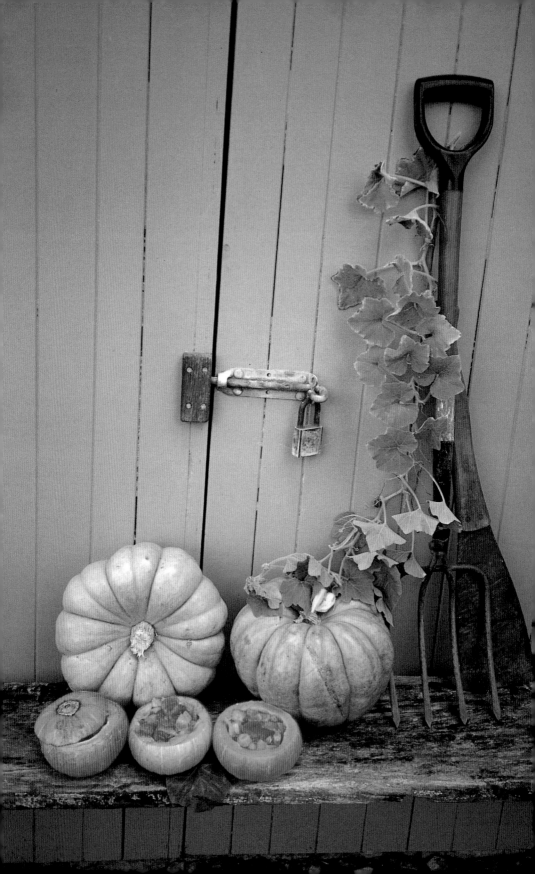

Mint Dressing

3 tabs mint, chopped finely
1 clove garlic, crushed
½ cup no-oil French dressing (page 111)
2 tabs lemon juice

Combine ingredients in a screw top jar, shake well.

Dill and Lime Dressing

2 tabs lime juice
1 tabs no-oil Italian dressing (page 111)
2 tabs chopped fresh dill

Combine ingredients in a screw-top jar, shake well.

Basic White Sauce

2 teas non fat-dry powdered milk
1½ cups non-fat skim milk
1 tabs cornflour (blended with ¼ cup milk)
1 teas soy sauce, low salt
black pepper

Blend powdered milk and skim milk together. Place milk in saucepan and bring to boil. Blend cornflour with a little milk and mix to a smooth paste. Add to simmering milk. Add soy sauce and pepper and stir constantly until thickened.

Mustard Yoghurt Dressing

½ cup natural yoghurt
2 tabs lime juice
2 teas Dijon mustard
1 clove garlic, crushed
snipped chives

Mix ingredients together.

LEFT: *Stuffed Golden Nugget Pumpkins (page 134)*

Thousand Island Dressing

1 cup mock sour cream (page 112)
2 drops Worcestershire sauce
¼ teas finely grated onion
1 finely chopped hard boiled egg white (optional)
1 tabs tomato paste (unsalted)
dash black pepper
2 teas finely chopped parsley

Combine all ingredients and mix well. Thin the dressing with skim milk if necessary. For a sharper taste, lemon juice can be added.

Apple Juice Salad Dressing

2 cups unsweetened apple juice
pinch black pepper
½ teas garlic powder
½ cup cider vinegar
2 teas chopped parsley

Mix ingredients together, put in an airtight bottle and shake well. Store in refrigerator. Serve with salad.

Lemon and Garlic Dressing

1 cup lemon juice
2 cloves garlic, crushed

Mix well together and serve over salad.

Herb Dressing

½ cup no-oil French dressing (page 111)
1 tabs chives, chopped
2 cloves garlic, crushed
1 tabs fresh dill, chopped
1 tabs mint, chopped
1 tabs each fresh coriander and fresh basil, chopped

Combine all ingredients in a screw-top jar, shake well.

Low-fat Mayonnaise

½ cup skim milk ricotta cheese (1% fat)
½ cup non-fat yoghurt
2 tabs water
2 teas lemon juice
1 tabs cider vinegar
½ teas dry mustard

Combine a little of the water with the yoghurt and cheese in a blender. Mix with vinegar, lemon juice and mustard to a smooth consistency. If too thick, thin out with more milk or water.

Tartare Mayonnaise

1½ cups low-fat mayonnaise (see above)
1 gherkin, chopped
1 teas capers, chopped
1 teas mixed herbs
hard boiled egg white, chopped
2 teas chopped parsley

Combine all ingredients together, chill and serve with fish dishes.

Goddess Mayonnaise

2 ripe avocados
pinch garlic powder
1 tabs lemon juice
2 teas mint, finely chopped

Mash the flesh of avocados with a silver spoon, press it through a sieve, mix with garlic powder and lemon juice, top with mint. May be thinned out with a little skim milk if too thick.

Sweet and Sour Sauce

¼ cup cider vinegar
1 tabs tomato paste (unsalted)
½ teas chopped green ginger (or ground ginger)
¼ cup apple juice

1 tabs sherry
3/4 cup pineapple juice

Combine all ingredients.

Tomato Sauce

14 peeled ripe tomatoes
½ cup onions, chopped
2 garlic cloves, crushed
½ cup chopped celery with tops
¼ cup chopped parsley
¼ teas dried basil
juice of 2 lemons (optional)

Place the tomatoes in a saucepan with onions, garlic, celery, parsley and basil. Bring to boil, reduce heat and simmer for 30 minutes. Strain, return to saucepan and simmer uncovered for 1 hour or until thick. Makes 3 cups.

Del's Eezee Tomato Sauce

4 tabs tomato paste (unsalted)
2 cups unsweetened tomato juice
½ teas onion powder
½ teas garlic powder or small clove freshly crushed garlic
herbs of your choice (just a pinch!)—sweet basil, parsley,
    rosemary, thyme, sage, oregano

Mix ingredients, simmer over gentle heat until boiling. Boil very gently for a minute or two. Cool, pour into container. Store in refrigerator. Make up small quantities and use within a day or two, as this is free of preservatives and its keeping life is limited.

Dad's Spaghetti Sauce

400 g (14 oz) can tomatoes (unsalted)
½ cup tomato paste (unsalted)
2 onions, chopped
3 garlic cloves, crushed

1 teas oregano
black pepper
2 teas soy sauce, low salt
2 tabs water

Chop tomatoes. In a saucepan add tomatoes, tomato paste, onions, garlic, oregano, a good pinch of pepper, soy sauce and water, bring to boil and simmer for 15 minutes. Makes 2 cups. Serve with wholemeal spaghetti.

Chinese Sauce

6 water chestnuts, finely chopped
1 teas soy sauce
1 tabs sherry
1 cup chicken stock
1 tabs honey
1 teas ginger, chopped
1 clove garlic, crushed
dash black pepper
1 tabs cornflour

Blend all ingredients together. Cook in a non-stick frypan, stirring constantly, for about 5 minutes. Add water to thin if too thick. Serve over rice or vegetables.

Tomato Garlic Sauce

½ cup tomato juice, unsalted
2 garlic cloves, crushed
½ cup cider vinegar
¼ cup green pepper, finely chopped
2 tabs onions, finely chopped
1 teas cumin

Combine all ingredients, place in a saucepan and bring to boil. Simmer for 10 minutes, stirring occasionally. Makes 2 cups.

Salads

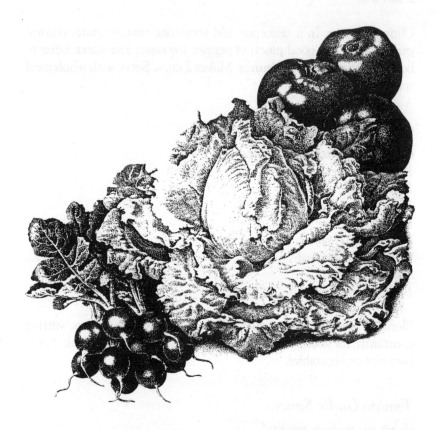

In America one can find soup and salad bars all over. People should be aware that salad can be a meal by itself—it should not be regarded purely as an accessory.

A crisp, fresh delicious salad arranged on a large oval dish is very appealing to the eye and palate. Serve with hot thick soup and crusty bread and you will enjoy a very nourishing meal low in kilojoules. Lemon juice with crushed garlic is a good dressing with no kilojoules. This dressing adds a sharp tang to salads and steamed vegetables.

Mandarin Coleslaw

½ cabbage, shredded
½ onion, chopped
2 carrots, grated
2 mandarins, peeled and segmented
1 tabs coriander, chopped

Dressing

1 cup low-fat mayonnaise (page 115)
¼ cup raw honey
½ cup orange juice
1 teas mixed dry mustard

Combine cabbage, onion, carrot and mandarin segments together, mix
with dressing.

Avocado Lime Salad

1 mignonette lettuce, torn
1 large avocado, chopped
1 small green pepper, chopped
1 small red pepper, chopped
2 shallots, chopped
1 tabs parsley, chopped

Dressing

½ cup no-oil French dressing (page 111)
¼ cup lime juice
1 garlic clove, crushed
1 tabs tarragon, fresh
1 tabs coriander, fresh
black pepper

Arrange lettuce leaves on a platter, mix remaining ingredients together
with dressing, place on top of lettuce, sprinkle with parsley.

Mango and Pine Nut Salad

1 cos lettuce
1 mango, chopped
¼ cup pine nuts
½ cup no-oil French dressing (page 111)
black pepper

Toast pine nuts on a non-stick baking tray about 6 minutes until golden, cool. Break lettuce leaves into pieces, arrange pine nuts and mango on top of lettuce. Pour French dressing over salad.

Cucumber and Mint Tomatoes

4 Lebanese cucumbers, peeled and diced
2 large tomatoes, chopped
2 shallots, chopped
1 tabs mint, chopped
1 garlic clove, crushed
black pepper

Dressing
½ cup no-oil French dressing (page 111)
¼ cup lime juice

Toss salad ingredients together, combine lime juice and dressing, mix with salad ingredients.

Stuffed Lettuce Leaves

18 large lettuce leaves
no-oil French dressing (page 111)
¼ cup lemon juice
black pepper

Filling
1 avocado
2 stalks celery, finely chopped

1 small onion, finely chopped
½ cup mock sour cream (page 112)

Cut lettuce leaves into 5 cm (2") strips, place in a bowl with French dressing and lemon juice, grind black pepper over leaves.
Mash avocado flesh with a fork, combine with celery, onion and sour cream, place on lettuce leaves, roll up and secure with a toothpick.

Carrot and Raisin Salad

4 large carrots, grated
1 cup raisins
½ cup orange juice
¼ cup no-oil French dressing (page 111)

Mix all ingredients together.

Mexican Salad

1 lettuce
1 red onion, sliced
1 orange, pithed and peeled
1 grapefruit, pithed and peeled
½ cup cherry tomatoes
1 avocado, peeled and sliced
1 corn cob (steamed and peeled)
½ can kidney beans (no salt)
parsley
black pepper

Dressing
½ cup no-oil French dressing (page 111)
¼ cup fresh lime juice
1 garlic clove, crushed
1 teas ground cumin
½ teas red chilli, crushed (optional)

Combine dressing ingredients. Place lettuce leaves on a platter, arrange onion rings on top, add orange and grapefruit segments, top with tomatoes, avocado, corn kernels and kidney beans, sprinkle with parsley and pepper. Pour over dressing.

Pear Salad

4 ripe pears, halved
lettuce leaves
½ cup ricotta cheese
lemon juice

Fill each pear half with ricotta cheese, sprinkle with lemon juice. Arrange on lettuce leaves.

Green Salad

½ cos lettuce, torn
10 small spinach leaves, torn
½ romaine lettuce, torn
sprigs of snow pea sprouts
sprigs of watercress
sprigs of dill
1 onion, chopped
1 garlic clove, crushed
2 tabs coriander
a few yellow marigold petals
1 lime, sliced thinly
2 tabs parsley
black pepper

Dressing
1 cup no-oil French dressing (page 111)
1 tabs fresh lime juice
1 tabs melted raw honey

Combine dressing ingredients. Mix salad greens together, pour over dressing.

122

Watermelon Salad

½ watermelon, seeded and balled
3 large tomatoes, sliced thinly
1 red onion, peeled and sliced
1 Lebanese cucumber, sliced thinly

Dressing
¼ cup no-oil French dressing (page 111)
¼ cup lemon juice
1 tabs melted raw honey

Combine dressing ingredients. Edge salad platter with tomato slices, arrange watermelon balls, onion rings and cucumber in centre. Pour over dressing.

Rice Salad

½ cup brown rice
½ cup Basmati rice
¼ cup pine nuts
2 corn cobs
½ cup dried apricots, halved
½ cup dried figs, halved

Dressing
½ cup no-oil French dressing (page 111)
2 tabs lemon juice
1 teas cinnamon

Combine dressing ingredients. Boil brown rice for 20 minutes, add white rice, boil a further 10 minutes or until tender. Drain and cool. Cook corn for 15 minutes, strip corn off cobs. Meanwhile toast pine nuts on a non-stick baking tray for 6 minutes until golden. Add corn, apricots and figs to rice, mix with dressing and sprinkle with pine nuts.

Gazpacho Salad

2 medium Lebanese cucumbers, peeled and thinly sliced
1 large onion, sliced
2 large tomatoes, sliced
10 medium mushrooms, sliced
1 small green pepper, slivered
8 slices non-fat cheese
black pepper
1 tabs oregano, fresh

Dressing
½ cup no-oil French dressing (page 111)
1 garlic clove, crushed
1 teas basil

Combine dressing ingredients. Mix cucumber, onion, add dressing, top mixture with sliced tomatoes, mushroom and green pepper. Top with cheese, sprinkle with pepper and oregano.

Cucumber Salad with Avocado Dill Dressing

3 Lebanese cucumbers, thinly sliced
1 cup watercress sprigs, chopped
fresh dill sprigs

Dressing
1 avocado, peeled and seeded
½ cup low-fat mayonnaise (page 115)
1 tabs lemon juice

Mash avocado with fork, combine with lemon juice and mayonnaise to make dressing. Combine cucumber and watercress, mix with dressing. Garnish with dill.

Orange Salad

4 oranges
1 red onion, sliced
watercress sprigs

Dressing
¼ cup no-oil French dressing (page 111)
¼ cup orange juice
1 teas grated orange rind

Peel oranges, remove pith, peel into segments, combine with onion and watercress. Arrange in a bowl, pour over dressing.

Waldorf Salad

1 cos lettuce (torn into pieces)
1 cup finely chopped celery chunks
1 cup finely chopped apple chunks
½ cup walnuts
fresh chives, snipped
black pepper

Dressing
1 cup low-fat mayonnaise (page 115)
½ teas prepared mustard powder
1 tabs melted raw honey

Combine dressing ingredients. Arrange salad ingredients in a bowl, mix with dressing. Garnish with chives and black pepper.

Zucchini Coleslaw

6 large zucchinis
2 cups water
½ cup low-fat mayonnaise (page 115)
2 onions, peeled and finely chopped
1 tabs parsley, chopped

2 teas Dijon mustard
1 punnet cherry tomatoes
½ cabbage, finely chopped

Cut off zucchini ends, bring water to boil, add zucchini, simmer 10 minutes or until tender. Drain. Cut zucchini lengthwise into quarters. Combine mayonnaise, onion, parsley and mustard, pour over zucchini, marinade chilled for 2 hours. Divide zucchini into 4 portions and garnish with tomatoes. Arrange on the cabbage. Pour marinade dressing over each serving.

Salad Kebabs

½ lettuce
1 onion
1 green pepper
1 red pepper
1 cucumber
no-fat cheese
1 punnet cherry tomatoes
8 tabs salad dressing

Cut onion, peppers, cucumber and cheese into 16 chunks. Arrange with tomatoes onto 8 wooden kebab sticks. Place lettuce leaves on a long slim salad platter. Top with kebabs. Add a spoonful of your favourite salad dressing to each kebab.

Pea and Tomato Salad

1 cucumber
2 cups fresh peas
1 punnet cherry tomatoes
4 shallots, chopped

Dressing

½ cup no-oil French dressing (page 111)
2 tabs chopped mint
1 garlic clove, crushed

Combine dressing ingredients. Cut cucumber in half lengthwise, remove seeds, slice thinly. Combine cucumber, peas, quartered tomatoes and shallots in a bowl. Mix with dressing. Serves 4.

Avocado and Grapefruit Salad

1 medium avocado
1 grapefruit
1 small lettuce
chives, snipped
black pepper

Dressing
½ cup no-oil French dressing (page 111)
¼ cup lemon juice
1 garlic clove, crushed

Peel, stone and slice avocado. Peel and pith grapefruit, divide into segments. Place 4 lettuce leaves on each plate, arrange avocado and grapefruit alternately on lettuce. Pour over dressing, garnish with chives and black pepper. Serves 4.

Salad Nicoise

4 eggs
can artichokes
1 small red pepper, sliced into fine slivers
500 g (1 lb) fresh broad beans
1 small cucumber, thinly sliced
2 large tomatoes (cut into eighths)
2 celery stalks, cut into thin strips
2 shallots, chopped
1 garlic clove
12 anchovy fillets
1 small can no-salt tuna, drained
12 black olives
½ cup no-oil French dressing (page 111)
parsley
black pepper

Boil eggs for 10 minutes, cool, shell and scoop out yolks. Use only the whites. Cut into slices. Shell the broad beans and remove the green outer skins. Remove the outer leaves of artichokes, cut into quarters and rub with lemon. Rub salad bowl with garlic clove. Arrange remaining salad ingredients in bowl. Garnish with anchovies, tuna, olives and eggs, sprinkle with dressing and parsley. Serves 4.

Potato and Coriander Salad

4 large potatoes
2 cups water
2 carrots, peeled and grated
1 red pepper, seeded and slivered
1 onion, grated
1 cup low-fat mayonnaise (page 115)
3 tabs coriander, chopped
black pepper

Peel and chop potatoes, bring to the boil, reduce heat and simmer until tender. Drain and cool. Add remaining ingredients. Mix with mayonnaise. Garnish with coriander and black pepper. Serves 4.

Sesame Beans

1 bunch green snake beans
2 tabs sesame seeds, toasted

Dressing
¼ cup lemon juice
¼ cup no-oil French dressing (page 111)
2 tabs honey

Trim beans, cook for 5 minutes in steamer, cool. Pour over dressing and sprinkle with sesame seeds. Serves 4.

RIGHT: Food by the pool, featuring Two-tone Green and White Soup (page 103) and Coconut Cream Soup with Prawns (page 100), decorated with crabs and other seafood

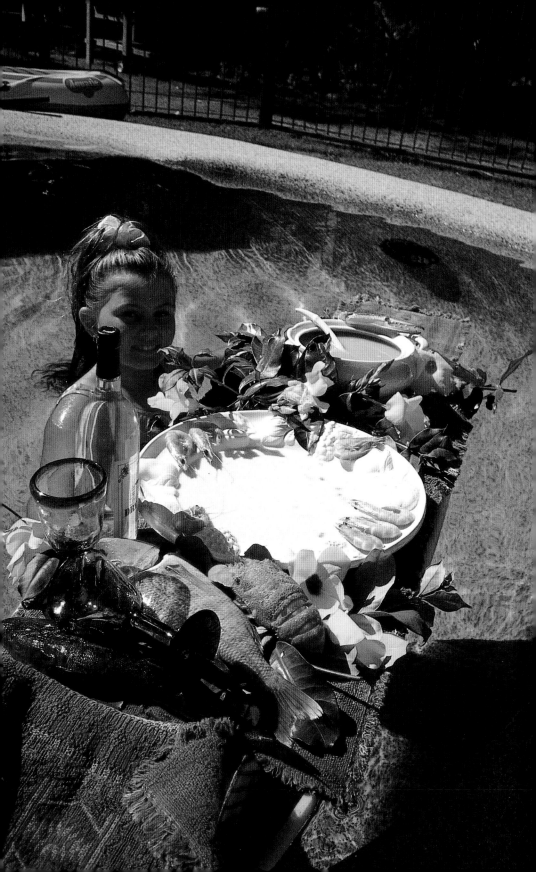

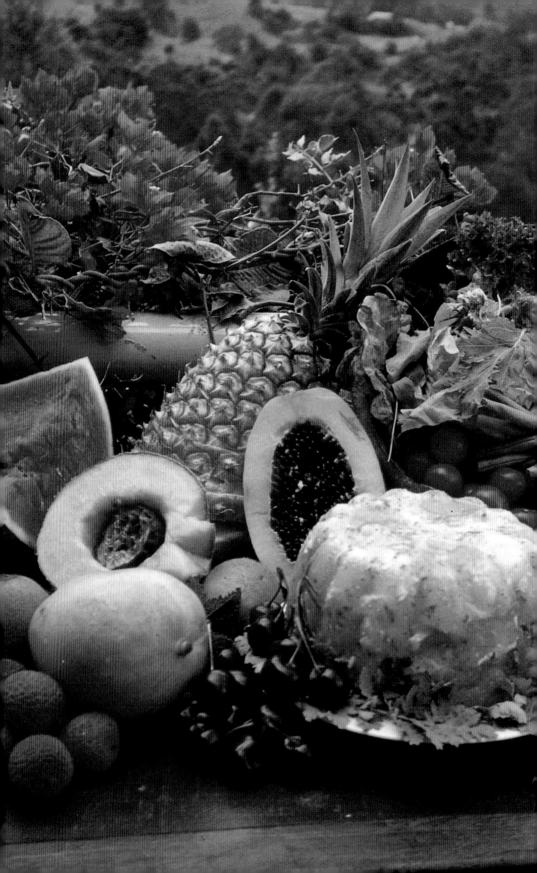

Special Salad

1 lettuce, torn into pieces
1 cup bean sprouts
1 tomato, chopped and diced
½ Lebanese cucumber, sliced
2 carrots, grated
½ cup cauliflower flowerets
½ cup celery, chopped
½ green pepper, chopped

Dressing

½ cup lemon juice
garlic clove, crushed

Combine lemon juice and garlic. Mix salad ingredients, toss in garlic dressing. Serves 4.

Millionaire's Salad

1 lettuce
1 bunch asparagus, steamed
2 carrots, peeled and cut into fine strips
10 green beans, sliced finely
can artichoke hearts
1 cucumber, peeled and sliced finely
1 large avocado, peeled, stoned and sliced
1 punnet cherry tomatoes
6 radishes
3 shallots, chopped finely

Crabmeat Dressing

1 cup low-fat mayonnaise (page 115)
juice 1 lemon
250 g (8 oz) crabmeat
3 hard boiled eggs (whites only), chopped

LEFT: A bougainvillea-draped terrace forms a background for Chicken Terrine (page 150), with a platter of tropical fruit and Millionaire's Salad (opposite)

Mix dressing ingredients. Arrange salad vegetables on a bed of lettuce on a large platter. Serve dressing in a bowl in the centre of the platter. Serves 4.

Moulded Gazpacho with Avocado Dressing

2 small tomatoes, peeled and diced
1 medium cucumber, peeled and sliced
½ medium red pepper, seeded and diced
1 tabs onion, chopped
1 tabs chives, chopped
¼ cup celery, chopped
2 envelopes gelatine
3 cups tomato juice

Avocado Dressing

1 ripe avocado, mashed
1 tabs lemon juice
1 cup low-fat mayonnaise (page 115)
1 clove garlic, crushed
black pepper

Combine dressing ingredients. Sprinkle gelatine over tomato juice and stir over low heat until dissolved. Remove from heat. Stir. Chill until practically set. Add vegetables and stir. Pour into mould. Set and unmould. Serve with avocado dressing. Serves 4.

The Lakes Delight

1 cos lettuce, torn into pieces
½ bunch small spinach leaves
1 mignonette lettuce
a few marigold petals
1 avocado, stoned, peeled and chopped into pieces
2 tomatoes, chopped
1 Lebanese cucumber, chopped
½ bottle small anchovy fillets
125 g (4 oz) ricotta cheese, cut into chunks

¼ *cup pine nuts*
sprig of dill, black pepper

Dressing
½ *cup no-oil French dressing (page 111)*
½ *teas mixed dry mustard*

Combine French dressing and mustard. Spread pine nuts on a non-stick baking tray and toast in oven for 6 minutes or until golden. Line an oval serving platter with green salad ingredients. Arrange avocado, tomatoes, cucumber, anchovies and ricotta cheese. Sprinkle with pine nuts and black pepper, garnish with dill. Serves 4.

Asparagus Parmesan

1 bunch asparagus
6 shallots, diagonally sliced
¼ *cup lemon juice*
1 tabs cider vinegar
1 teas fresh ginger grated
¼ *cup sesame seeds*
freshly grated parmesan cheese

Spread sesame seeds on a non-stick baking tray and toast for 6 minutes or until golden. Steam asparagus until just tender. Cool. Combine asparagus and shallots. Mix lemon juice, vinegar and ginger, pour over asparagus. Sprinkle parmesan and sesame seeds over asparagus. Serves 4.

Fruit Ricotta

125 g (4 oz) ricotta cheese
lettuce, torn into pieces
1 apple, chopped
1 kiwi fruit, peeled and chopped
4 walnuts, halved

Arrange lettuce leaves, apple, kiwi fruit on a plate. Place cheese in middle and sprinkle with walnuts. Serves 4.

Manhattan Caesar Salad

1 cos lettuce, torn and chilled
½ cup freshly grated parmesan cheese
½ cup croutons

Dressing
¼ cup fresh lemon juice
⅓ cup red wine vinegar
⅔ cup no-oil French dressing (page 111)
1 large anchovy fillet
garlic, crushed to taste
black pepper
dash of Worcestershire sauce
1 egg white, lightly beaten

Blend together lemon juice, vinegar and oil. Set aside. In another small bowl mash anchovy to a paste, add garlic, pepper and Worcestershire sauce. Add egg white and mix well, then beat in lemon juice mixture until thoroughly blended.

Pour desired amount of dressing over lettuce and croutons a little at a time. Sprinkle with parmesan cheese. Serves 4.

Main Course Dishes

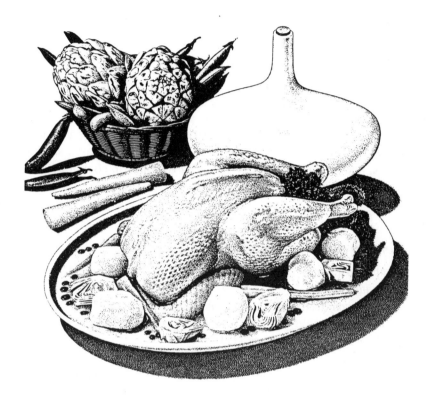

Chinese Vegetables with Sweet Curry Sauce

½ cup almonds, slivered and toasted
½ cup celery, sliced diagonally
½ medium red pepper, seeded and cut into thin strips
½ medium green pepper, seeded and cut into thin strips
1 onion, cut into eighths
½ cup shallots, chopped
1 cup bean shoots
½ cup stock or water
1 teas soy sauce, low salt

In a non-stick frypan or wok add stock, vegetables and soy sauce, cook until tender. Do not overcook. Mix in almonds.

133

Sweet Curry Sauce
1 onion, finely chopped
1 clove garlic, crushed
2 teas cornflour
2 cups stock
2 teas curry powder
1 tabs chutney
½ cup sultanas
1 apple, peeled and chopped

In a non-stick pan saute onion and garlic in a little water, add stock, blend cornflour with a little water to make a smooth paste, stir into stock, add remaining ingredients, bring to boil, stir, cook for 5 minutes. Serve with vegetables. Serves 2.

Tomato and Onion Surprise

1 cup breadcrumbs
3 tomatoes, sliced
1 small onion, sliced and separated into rings
2 tabs snipped chives
1 cup mock sour cream (page 112)

Line a non-stick casserole dish with half the breadcrumbs. Alternate tomato and onion slices. Mix chives with sour cream, spread over tomato and onion rings. Sprinkle with remaining breadcrumbs. Bake uncovered in a moderate oven for 45 minutes or until lightly browned and cooked through. Serves 4.

Stuffed Nugget Pumpkins

4 nugget pumpkins
2 onions, chopped
2 cloves garlic, crushed
3 large tomatoes, chopped
½ teas chilli powder
2 teas cumin
2 tabs tomato paste
½ cup white wine

Cut 3 cm (1¼") lid from each pumpkin, scoop out seeds, place pumpkin with lid on oven tray. Bake for 50 minutes in moderate oven until cooked. Saute onions, garlic, tomatoes in a non-stick pan, add chilli powder, cumin, tomato paste and wine. Cook 10 minutes, pile into pumpkin shells. Serves 4.

Spinach Ricotta Burgers

½ bunch spinach leaves
3 carrots, grated
1 cup ricotta cheese
parsley
½ cup ground almonds
½ cup dried breadcrumbs
tamari to taste

Combine all ingredients except almonds and crumbs. Mix well and form into burger shapes. Roll in breadcrumbs and almonds. Bake the burgers on a non-stick baking tray for about 20 minutes or until cooked.

Serve with salad or steamed vegetables. Also excellent for lunch as a pita and sandwich filling.

Sunshine Corn Casserole

1 medium onion, chopped
6 yellow squash, sliced
1 clove garlic, crushed
1 teas ground cumin
black pepper
2 cups corn kernels
1 cup grated cheese, non-fat
breadcrumbs

Saute onion in a little water in a non-stick frypan, add squash, cover and steam until squash is tender. Drain and add seasonings and corn. Cover and cook 5 minutes more. Stir in cheese and place in a casserole dish, top with breadcrumbs. Bake at 175°C (350°F) for 25 to 30 minutes. Serve with salad. Serves 4.

135

Oriental Peas with Onion Rings

2 cups cooked green peas
½ cup sliced water chestnuts
½ cup fresh bean sprouts
12 mushrooms, sauteed
soy sauce (no salt), to taste
2 onions, sliced into rings

White Sauce
1 cup skim milk
½ cup mock sour cream (page 112)
1 teas cornflour
black pepper

Heat milk and sour cream together, do not boil. Stir in cornflour mixed with a little water to thicken, add pepper. Mix sauce through the remaining ingredients (except onion rings). Bake at 175°C (350°F) for 30 minutes. Top with onion rings and bake 10 minutes more. Serve with salad. Serves 4.

Vine Leaf Parcels with Rich Mango Sauce

250 g (4 oz) vine leaves (about 30)
½ cup rice
6 shallots, chopped
2 tabs pine nuts, chopped
1 tabs parsley, chopped
2 tabs mint, chopped
1 cup stock or water
1 lemon for juice
1 lemon, sliced

Saute chopped shallots, pine nuts and rice in a non-stick frypan. Cook for 5 minutes, stirring. Add parsley, mint and stock, cover and bring to boil. Reduce heat, cook for another 10 minutes or until water is absorbed. In the meantime, blanch vine leaves. Rinse, cool, and pat dry. Place a teaspoonful of rice mixture in each vine leaf (shiny side out) and roll up-not too tightly as rice will expand. Make rows of vine leaves in a saucepan. Squeeze juice of 1 lemon over and add enough water to cover rolls.

Place a plate on the rolls to weigh them down, cover saucepan with lid and cook for about 1½ hours. Cool in saucepan.

Mango Sauce
1 large mango
½ cup mock sour cream (page 112)

Combine sauce ingredients in a blender for 1 minute. Arrange vine leaf parcels on a serving dish on a bed of fresh grape leaves. Garnish with lemon slices and fresh dill and serve with the chilled mango sauce.

Cabbage and Rice Rolls in Tomato Sauce
8 cabbage leaves
1 cup rice, cooked
4 shallots, chopped
1 clove garlic, crushed
1 cup ricotta cheese, crumbled

Cook cabbage leaves in a little water until soft, drain. Boil rice in a large saucepan of water about 10 minutes until soft. Drain and wash under tap to separate grains. Combine rice with remaining ingredients, divide between cabbage leaves, roll up, tucking in ends, place in a single layer on a shallow overproof dish.

Tomato Sauce
1 clove garlic, crushed
1 small onion, chopped
2 medium ripe tomatoes, peeled and chopped
½ cup chicken stock
¼ cup white wine
fresh oregano, chopped

Saute garlic and onion in a little water in a non-stick frypan, stir until onion is soft, add remaining ingredients and cook for about 10 minutes. Pour over cabbage rolls, cover and bake in a medium oven for 30 minutes. Serves 4.

Crunchy Oatmeal and Kumara Bake

3 cups mashed kumara (orange sweet potato
1 cup mashed squash
1 cup skim milk
1 tabs lemon juice
1 teas grated lemon rind
1 teas allspice
1 teas ground ginger
3 egg whites, stiffly beaten
2/3 cup rolled oats

Combine kumara, squash and milk. Add lemon juice, rind and spices. Blend egg whites into potato mixture.

Soak oatmeal quickly in cold water to soften, then place in the bottom of a non-stick baking pan or foil-lined pan. Bake in 175°C (350°F) oven for 15 minutes or until the oatmeal layer is browned and dry. Fill pan with kumara mixture. Bake for 30 minutes at same temperature. Serve with salad. Serves 4.

Tantalising Parsnip Souffle

3 cups cooked mashed parsnips
1 cup skim milk
2 teas cornflour
1 teas nutmeg
cayenne pepper, pinch
2 egg whites
½ cup stale breadcrumbs
½ cup low-fat cheese, grated
paprika

Warm milk, thicken with cornflour mixed with a little water to a smooth paste. Add cooked mashed parsnips and spices. Beat egg whites stiffly till peaks form. Fold gently into parsnip mixture. Place into a casserole dish, top with breadcrumbs and sprinkle with cheese and paprika. Bake 30 minutes in a moderate oven. Serve with salad. Serves 4.

Prawn-stuffed Zucchini

8 large zucchinis

Filling
175 g (6 oz) green prawns, peeled
10 mushrooms, sliced
½ cup breadcrumbs
½ cup low-fat cheese, grated

Boil zucchini until tender, set aside. Saute prawns until they turn red, add mushrooms, cook 3 minutes. Mix in breadcrumbs and cheese. Slice zucchinis lengthwise, scrape out pulp, stuff with filling. Serves 4.

Baked Eggplant with Cheese Sauce

2 large eggplants
1 large onion, chopped
3 tomatoes, chopped
1 teas ground basil
1 tabs parsley, chopped
black pepper
1 teas soy sauce, low-salt
3/4 cup cottage cheese, non-fat
2 tabs milk
2 tabs stale breadcrumbs

Wash eggplants, don't peel. Cut into 2 cm (1") slices, brown in a non-stick frypan. Set aside slices. In same pan in a little water saute onion, tomatoes, basil, parsley, pepper and soy sauce for about 10 minutes. Blend cottage cheese and milk together. Divide egg plant slices into three portions. Place one portion in the base of a casserole, top with half tomato mixture and spread half cheese sauce on top of tomato. Place on more eggplant slices, then remaining tomato mixture and cheese sauce. Finish with layer of eggplant and top with breadcrumbs. Bake at 175°C (350°F) for about 20 minutes. Serves 4.

Stuffed Minty Zucchini

4 large zucchini
1 medium onion, chopped
½ cup cooked brown rice
4 tabs mint, chopped
nutmeg
black pepper
1 cup tomato puree

Cook zucchini in boiling water for 5 minutes until tender. Split in half lengthwise and scoop out pulp, chop pulp into pieces. Saute onion in a little water and add to rice, mint, pepper, nutmeg, ½ cup tomato puree and zucchini pulp. Mix well and spoon into zucchini shells. Place stuffed zucchini in a shallow non-stick or foil-lined casserole dish, pour remaining tomato puree around zucchini, cover and bake at 175°C (350°F) for 30 minutes. Serves 4.

Gnocchi

3 large potatoes, peeled and diced
1 cup steamed spinach, chopped
125 grams ricotta cheese, crumbled
2 tabs chives, snipped
½ cup plain flour
tomato sauce (page 116)

Boil potatoes until tender, drain, process in blender. Knead ricotta cheese, chives and spinach into potato mixture, work in sifted flour. Turn onto a floured surface, knead until smooth. Roll dough into small balls. Make indentations in balls with a fork. Bring large saucepan of water to the boil, add half the balls, reduce heat and simmer for 5 minutes or until balls float to the top. Remove, keep warm, repeat with remaining balls. Serve with tomato sauce. Serves 4.

Herbed Capanato with Pasta

2 onions, chopped
2 garlic cloves, crushed
1 eggplant, chopped into cubes

3 large tomatoes, peeled and chopped
1 tabs fresh basil
300 g (12 oz) pasta

In a non-stick pan saute onion and garlic in a little water. Add egg-plant, tomatoes and basil and cook for 5 minutes. Cook pasta in large pan of boiling water and boil uncovered until al dente. Drain and rinse with warm water. Serve with capanato sauce. Serves 4.

Linguini with White Scallop Sauce

3 large onions, chopped
4 cloves garlic, crushed
500 g (1 lb) sea scallops (prawns may be used instead)
½ cup fish stock or water
½ cup white wine
ground black pepper
3 tabs lemon juice
500 g (1 lb) linguini (angel-hair pasta), cooked and drained

Saute onions and garlic with a little water in a non-stick frypan until onions have softened. Add scallops, stock, wine, pepper and lemon juice. Cook about 8 minutes until scallops are tender. Serve over linguini with side salad. Serves 4.

Wholemeal Lasagna with Cheese Sauce

500 g (1 lb) wholemeal lasagna noodles
2 potatoes, peeled and thinly sliced
1 green pepper, sliced
2 carrots, grated
2 cups Dad's Spaghetti Sauce (page 116)
3 cups low-fat cottage cheese
2 egg whites
2 teas parsley

Mix cottage cheese, egg whites and parsley together to make cheese mixture. Cook lasagne noodles according to instructions. Place a thin layer of spaghetti sauce on bottom of a casserole dish. Place a layer of the drained noodles over this, then layer some grated carrots, some potatoes, some green pepper, then a layer of cheese mixture, then more spaghetti sauce. Repeat this sequence, building up several noodle layers, and end with sauce. Bake in 190°C (370°F) oven for 35 minutes or until set. Sprinkle with parsley. Serves 4.

Milano Fish Balls with Pasta

¼ cabbage, about 2 cups
500 g (1 lb) gem fish (or any other white fish)
2 tabs shallots, finely chopped
2 egg whites, beaten
2 garlic cloves, crushed
3 tabs red pepper, finely chopped
2 large tomatoes, peeled and chopped
1 tabs tomato paste
2 teas oregano
250 g (8 oz) pasta
parmesan cheese
parsley

Cook cabbage in a little water until soft, drain and chop. Blend fish in a food processor until smooth, add to shallots, egg whites, cabbage. Shape into balls. Combine red pepper, tomatoes, tomato paste, oregano in a saucepan, bring to boil, reduce heat and simmer for 10 minutes. Add fish balls, cook further 15 minutes.

To a boiling saucepan of water add pasta. Cook until tender, about 10 minutes. Serve sauce over hot pasta, garnish with grated parmesan cheese and parsley.

Hungarian Ricotta and Spinach Dumplings

10 spinach leaves
1½ cups ricotta cheese
2 tabs grated parmesan cheese
1 egg white beaten
pinch of allspice

1½ tabs plain flour
sweet and sour sauce (page 115)

Steam spinach leaves until tender, drain well and chop finely. Combine with ricotta cheese, parmesan, egg and allspice, mix well. Roll into 10 balls. Dust with flour. Place balls gently into a large saucepan of boiling water, reduce heat, simmer for about 3 minutes until balls rise to the surface. Remove and drain, serve with sweet and sour sauce. Serves 2.

Indonesian Melange and Almond Rice

1 green pepper, cut into strips
1 large can pineapple chunks in juice, unsweetened
2 large tomatoes, peeled and cut into eighths
2 apples, peeled, cored and sliced
1 large banana
1 cup rice
3 tabs almonds
2 tabs parsley chopped

Sweet and Sour Sauce
½ cup pineapple juice, from the pineapple chunks
¼ cup wine vinegar
2 tabs honey
1 tabs soy sauce, low-salt
black pepper
1 teas cornflour
1 tabs water
cayenne pepper to taste

Combine pineapple juice, vinegar, honey, soy sauce and pepper in a saucepan. Mix cornflour with water. Heat the pineapple juice mixture and thicken with cornflour, cook over medium heat until thickened. Add cayenne pepper carefully. The sauce should be hot to taste with seasoning and temperature. Add fruits and vegetables and heat until they begin to soften, but are still crisp.

Boil rice for about 10 minutes until tender, wash under tap to separate grains. Toast almonds under grill for about 6 minutes, chop and mix with parsley through rice. Pour vegetables and sauce over rice. Serves 4.

Vegetable Paella Espana

1¼ cups brown rice
2 cups chicken stock
2 large onions, sliced
3 carrots, diced
3 zucchini, sliced thickly
2 cloves garlic
3 tomatoes
1 red pepper
1 green pepper
1 tabs tomato paste
½ teas turmeric
pepper
250 g (8 oz) broccoli, cut into flowerets

Parboil rice in stock for 15 minutes, set aside. Add onions, carrots, zucchini and crushed garlic to a non-stick frypan and cook about 10 minutes in 3 tabs water over medium heat. Add seeded and sliced peppers, tomato paste, turmeric and chopped tomatoes (peeled), cook for further 2 minutes. Add rice with stock and pepper (if desired) and stir until well combined with the rest. Simmer gently for further 15 minutes. Separately boil flowerets of broccoli for 3 minutes, drain and add to the rest. Arrange paella on serving plate and garnish with lemon wedges. Serves 4.

Cottage Cheese and Spinach Cannelloni

1 x 105 g (4 oz) packet cannelloni (15 tubes)
1 large onion, finely chopped
½ bunch cooked spinach or 250 g (8 oz) frozen spinach
2 garlic cloves, crushed
½ cup alfalfa sprouts
1 teas nutmeg
400 g (12 oz) non-fat cottage cheese

Tomato Sauce
400 g (12 oz) can tomatoes, unsalted
½ cup tomato paste, unsalted
1 large onion, finely chopped
2 garlic cloves, crushed
1 teas soy sauce, low fat
black pepper
½ cup water

Add cannelloni tubes to boiling water. Cook for 5 minutes, drain and set aside. In a saucepan cook spinach, onion and garlic in a little water for about 8 minutes. When cool, add cottage cheese, sprouts and nutmeg. Fill cannelloni tubes with mixture. Place tubes side by side in a non-stick baking dish. Combine sauce ingredients, cook in saucepan for 5 minutes. Pour sauce over cannelloni. Cover baking dish with foil and cook in 175°C (350°F) oven for 20 minutes. Garnish with parsley. Serves 4.

Avocado Gnocchi with Tomato Herb Sauce

2 avocados
4 tabs fresh parmesan cheese
250 g (8 oz) ricotta cheese
1 egg white
nutmeg
plain flour

Mash avocados with ricotta cheese, half the parmesan, egg white and nutmeg. Mix well and form into small balls. Roll lightly in flour. Bring a large pot of water to the boil and drop gnocchi in about 5 at a time. Simmer gently until the gnocchi rise to the surface-about 2 minutes. Remove with slotted spoon, sprinkle with remaining cheese and brown under grill.

Tomato Herb Sauce
2 large tomatoes, chopped
1 small onion, chopped
1 tabs basil, chopped
1 teas paprika

145

2 teas tomato paste, unsalted
1 bay leaf
1 tabs chopped parsley
1 clove garlic, crushed
¼ cup red wine
½ cup mock sour cream (page 112)

Mix all ingredients except sour cream together in a saucepan and cook for about 1 hour or until sauce is thick, stirring occasionally. Put through blender if a smooth sauce is preferred, but allow to cool a little first. Add sour cream just before serving and heat through. Pour over gnocchi.

Spicy Chicken and Mango Kebabs

2 chicken breasts, cubed
1 large mango, sliced

Marinade
1 garlic clove, crushed
2 teas fresh ginger, grated
2 tabs fresh coriander, chopped
½ cup lemon juice

Soak chicken in marinade overnight. Arrange chicken pieces alternately with mango slices on skewers. Grill, turning until chicken turns golden. Pour over mango sauce. Serve on a bed of rice with salad. Serves 4.

Mango Sauce
1 fresh mango, chopped
1 tabs fresh coriander, chopped
1 clove garlic, crushed
1 teas fresh ginger, grated
pinch chilli powder
pinch allspice
1 tabs honey

Blend ingredients together, heat if desired or serve cold.

Thai Chicken in Coconut Sauce

4 chicken breasts
2 tabs plain flour
½ cup coconut cream
fresh coriander to garnish

Coconut Sauce
1 small onion, finely chopped
2 cloves garlic, crushed
1 small fresh red chilli, finely chopped
1 tabs coriander root, chopped
1 tabs coriander leaves, chopped
1 teas ground cumin
1 tabs paprika
1 teas turmeric
¼ cup lime juice
1 teas grated lime rind

Toss chicken breasts in flour, brown in a non stick-pan. Stir coconut sauce ingredients together, add to chicken breasts, cook for about 10 minutes, stirring occasionally. Add coconut cream, simmer a further 10 minutes or until chicken is tender. Garnish with fresh coriander.

Special Spinach and Chicken Casserole

1 bunch spinach, washed and chopped
4 chicken breasts
2 tabs plain flour
1 onion, chopped
2 cloves garlic, crushed
1 cup chicken stock
½ cup mock sour cream (page 112)
½ cup white wine
parmesan cheese
1 tabs paprika

Steam spinach 5 minutes, chop and set aside. Toss chicken breasts in flour, brown in a non-stick pan, remove and set aside. To juices in pan add onion and garlic, cook 2 minutes. Add chicken stock, sour cream, wine and cook a further 2 minutes, stirring until blended. Line a casserole dish with spinach, arrange chicken breasts over spinach, pour sauce over chicken, sprinkle with parmesan cheese and paprika. Cover with foil, cook for 40 minutes in moderate oven, taking foil off for the last 10 minutes of cooking time to brown. Serve with salad and pasta. Serves 4.

Steamed Sesame Chicken with Snow Peas

4 chicken breasts
12 snow peas
2 tabs toasted sesame seeds

Sauce
½ cup coconut cream
½ cup white wine
1 tabs lemon juice
1 teas fresh ginger, grated
2 tabs coriander, chopped

Combine sauce ingredients. Steam chicken until tender, slice finely. Toast sesame seeds on oven tray in moderate oven about 6 minutes until golden. In the meantime steam snow peas 3 minutes. Place chicken on a serving plate, top with sauce, snow peas and sesame seeds. Serves 4.

Fruit-stuffed Chicken Breasts

1 cup apple, peeled and diced
1 cup pine nuts
½ cup raisins
1 can crushed pineapple, unsweetened
1 cup soft breadcrumbs, toasted
1 teas allspice
½ teas ground ginger
¼ teas ground cloves
6 chicken breasts

Reserve ½ cup drained pineapple and juice for sauce. Mix together remaining stuffing ingredients. Place 1/3 cup stuffing inside each breast. Fold over sides and fasten with skewers or string. Place chicken breasts in foil-lined or non-stick pan. Place pan in oven at 180°C (350°F) and bake for 30 minutes. Turn chicken and bake for 20 minutes more. Serve with fruit sauce.

Fruit Sauce
1 tabs honey
2 teas cornflour
1 teas allspice
½ teas ground ginger
1 cup orange juice
crushed pineapple and juice (reserved)
¼ cup raisins
slivered peel from orange
sections from one orange

Combine honey, cornflour, allspice and ginger and blend well. Mix in orange juice. Add reserved pineapple and juice and raisins. Cook and stir over medium heat until sauce comes to boil and thickens. Add orange sections and heat. Serves 6.

Chicken Breasts Salsa with Cajun Sauce

4 chicken breasts
2 tabs lemon juice
2 chillies, finely chopped
1 teas honey
2 tabs chopped fresh coriander
2 teas basil seed, toasted

Remove fat from chicken breasts and slice in half horizontally. Rub in lemon juice. In a non stick frypan add chillies, seeds as well, and cook in a little water. Add chicken and cook each side about 7 minutes or until tender. Add honey and coriander and sprinkle with basil seed. Serve with cajun sauce and salsa.

Cajun Sauce
½ tabs cayenne pepper
½ tabs fresh thyme, chopped
¼ cup parsley, chopped
1 teas soy sauce, low-salt
½ tabs black pepper
½ tabs fresh basil, chopped
1 tabs white pepper
1 cup ricotta cheese, blended

Combine all ingredients. Serve with chicken. Serves 4.

Salsa
corn, cut from 1 cob
1 large tomato
1 cucumber
2 tabs apple mint
1 tabs lemon juice

Remove seeds and dice peeled tomatoes and cucumber. Mix in corn, apple mint and lemon juice. Serve on the side.

Chicken Terrine
3 chicken breasts, cut in half
2 large onions, sliced
8 tabs chopped parsley
1 bay leaf
1 teas thyme
1 garlic clove, crushed
3 carrots
½ small lemon, sliced
1 cup white wine
3 envelopes gelatine
chives

Place chicken, onions, 6 tabs parsley, bay leaf, thyme, garlic, carrots and lemon in a pot with water to cover. Bring to boil, cover, reduce heat and simmer for 1 hour or until chicken is done. After first 20 minutes remove carrots, slice and save them. When chicken is done let it cool, remove skin and slice thinly. Scrape fat from stock and blend. Add 3 cups of stock to wine. Add gelatine and stir until dissolved. Chill until syrupy. Pour a thin layer of gelatine mixture into bottom of an 8-cup mould. Decorate with 3 lemon slices, 3 carrot slices and chives to form 3 flower sprays. Chill gelatine layer until firm, then fill mould with alternate layers of chicken and carrots. Combine the 2 tabs parsley with remaining gelatine stock mixture and pour into mould. Chill 4 hours. To unmould place in a bowl of hot water for 6 seconds. Serves 6.

Skewered Chicken with Pine Nut Honey Glaze

6 chicken thighs
½ cup pine nuts, chopped in blender

Honey Glaze
2 tabs honey
1 tabs soy sauce, low-salt
2 teas ginger, grated

Mix glaze ingredients in a saucepan, cook over low heat until honey is melted. Chop chicken into bite-size pieces, dip into glaze then roll into pine nuts. Thread on 8 skewers, leave overnight, barbecue or grill. Serve with salad. Serves 8.

Sashimi with Pink Pickled Ginger

250 g (8 oz) tuna fillet in one piece
chives
1 small cucumber
¼ giant white radish
pink Japanese ginger
watercress

Dip tuna into very hot water and then into dish of iced water to remove surface bacteria. Remove skin from tuna and cut diagonally to the grain, slicing as thinly as possible into narrow strips. Roll tuna up and tie with chives, forming bundles. Peel white radish, cut into 2.5 cm (1") cubes with a sharp knife to form a flower. On a large plate arrange sashimi rolls, decorate with radish flowers, pink ginger strips and watercress sprigs. Serve with dishes of soy sauce and horseradish.

Ginger Teriyaki Fish

4 white fish fillets
3 shallots, chopped
2 teas fresh ginger, grated
1 cup white wine
1 tabs teriyaki sauce
1 teas cornflour

Combine fish, shallots, ginger, wine and teriyaki sauce in a bowl, marinate overnight. Place ingredients in a non-stick pan, bring to boil, reduce heat, simmer until fish is tender. Remove fish, thicken sauce with cornflour mixed with a little water. Pour over fish before serving. Serves 4.

Fish Cutlets Steamed with Fresh Garden Herbs

4 fish cutlets (mackerel, blue-eyed cod or snapper)

Seasoning
2 cups stale white breadcrumbs
2 tabs fresh coriander, chopped
2 tabs parsley, chopped
2 tabs chives, chopped
1 tabs basil, chopped
2 tabs chutney
1 tabs garlic seeded mustard
1 egg white

Push a long sharp-bladed knife through the centre of each fillet lengthwise to make a pocket for stuffing. Combine seasoning ingredients, stuff the seasoning into the pocket of each fillet. Secure ends with tooth picks. Add a small amount of water to a large non-stick frypan. Cook fish over high heat for 5 minutes on either side. Serves 4.

Wine-baked Snapper

1 kg (2 lb) whole snapper
125 g (4 oz) mushrooms
1 medium onion
pepper
1 teas basil
1 egg white
1 cup fresh wholemeal bread crumbs
1 cup dry cooking wine
½ cup low-fat mayonnaise (see page 115)
½ cup mock sour cream (see page 112)
2 teas cornflour
4 shallots
2 tabs chopped parsley

Clean, scale and wash snapper, leaving head on; set aside. Place finely chopped mushrooms and onion in a non-stick frypan and cook gently until onion is soft. Add breadcrumbs, egg white, basil and pepper. Stuff this mixture into fish's cavity and sew up. Place fish in large baking dish, pour wine over. Cover dish with aluminium foil. Bake in 180°C (350°F) oven for 45 minutes or until fish is tender. Remove fish from dish, place on serving platter; keep warm.

Place baking dish on top of stove over medium heat, gradually stir in mayonnaise, sour cream, cornflour, chopped shallots and parsley. Stir until sauce boils and thickens. Reduce heat, simmer uncovered for 2 minutes. Serve sauce separately to pour over fish.

Fish is best served at table on large platter decorated with arrangement of vegetables of choice. Garnish with lemon wedges. Serves 4.

Fish Pie

1 cup white sauce (see page 113)
2 cups mashed potatoes
2 cups cooked flaked fish, cold
1 tabs grated onion
½ teas nutmeg
black pepper
1 tabs parsley
½ cup dry wholemeal breadcrumbs

Mix flaked fish, onion and parsley and place in pie dish. Cover with white sauce, add spices and top with potato mixture piped into rosettes. Sprinkle with breadcrumbs. Bake in oven at 200°C (400°F) for 25 minutes. Garnish with chopped parsley and lemon slices. Serves 4.

Fish Cutlets

4 fish cutlets
plain flour
black pepper
2 small onions, peeled and thinly sliced
1 clove garlic, crushed
125 g (4 oz) mushrooms, sliced
1 bay leaf
½ teas ground thyme
1 cup cider or white cooking wine
3 tabs non-fat yoghurt

In a non-stick baking dish place fish dredged in flour. Sprinkle with pepper and onion. Add garlic, mushrooms, bay leaf, thyme and cider. Cover and cook for 30 minutes in a moderate oven 190°C (375°F). Arrange fish cutlets on serving platter, remove bay leaf. Stir yoghurt into sauce remaining in baking dish. Garnish fish with capers and cover with sauce. Serves 4.

Fish Maitre d'Hotel

1 kg (2 lb) whole fish
4 shallots, chopped
½ cup white wine
1 cup white sauce (see page 113)
juice ½ lemon
1 tabs chopped parsley

Place fish in a casserole dish, sprinkle with pepper and shallots. Add wine, cover and cook in a slow oven at 160°C (325°F) for 15 minutes. Remove from oven, carefully drain off the liquid. Add liquid to the white sauce, lemon juice and parsley. Pour over fish, cover and continue cooking for further 15 minutes. Serve with lemon wedges or lemon and garlic dressing (see page 114). Serves 4.

Blue-eyed Cod with Creamy Avocado

4 blue-eyed cod cutlets
2 cloves garlic, crushed
1 onion, finely chopped

3 shallots, chopped
2 tabs lemon juice
½ glass white wine
1 teas cornflour

In a little water saute garlic, onion and shallots. Add cod, lemon juice and wine. Thicken with cornflour mixed with a little water. Cook fish for about 4 minutes on either side until tender.

Creamy Avocado
1 large avocado
1 jar black caviar
black pepper

Mash avocado with a fork until smooth. Shape into 4 balls. Arrange cod on individual serving plates, decorate each fillet with avocado ball and top with a teaspoon of caviar. Grind black pepper over.

Scallops Supreme Antonia

500 g (1 lb) fresh Tasmanian scallops
2 cloves garlic, crushed
1 onion, finely chopped
2 teas fresh ginger, grated
2 tabs coriander, chopped finely
1 tabs soy sauce
2 tabs plain flour
3/4 cup water or fish stock
juice of one lemon
2 tabs pine nuts, toasted
1 cup Basmati rice
1 cup diced green beans

In a little water saute garlic, onion and ginger, add coriander and soy sauce. Toss scallops in plain flour, add to onions with stock. Cook until scallops are tender, about 5 minutes. Meanwhile add rice to a large pot of boiling water, cook until tender. Steam beans for 5 minutes. Arrange boiled rice on a plate, top with beans. Pour over scallop mixture, squeeze lemon over scallops, sprinkle with pine nuts. Serve with sliced pawpaw and avocado. Serves 4.

Mango Lime Scallops with Pink Peppercorns

500 g (1 lb) sea scallops
3 shallots, chopped
¼ cup lime juice
1 teas grated lime rind
1 cup chicken stock
1 frozen or fresh mango, sliced
½ cup mock sour cream (see page 112)
fresh dill
4 tabs drained pink peppercorns

Saute shallots in a little water in a non-stick frypan until soft. Add scallops, lime juice, rind and chicken stock, cook for about 7 minutes until scallops are tender. Add mango slices and sour cream, just warmed. Serve on individual plates garnished with pink peppercorns and dill. Serve with rice. Serves 4.

Kiwi Whiting with Lemon Tarragon Sauce

4 fillets of whiting or other fish
1 tabs lemon juice
1 kiwi fruit
1 cup skim milk
1 tabs chopped parsley

Rub fish with lemon juice. Peel kiwi fruit and cut in 4 lengthwise. Place one piece of kiwi fruit across each piece of fish. Roll up and place in a shallow casserole. Pour over milk and bake at 180°C (350°F) for 10 minutes.

Lemon Tarragon Sauce

1 onion, chopped
½ cup chicken stock
1 teas cornflour
1/3 cup lemon juice
2 teas tarragon, chopped
1 tabs mock sour cream (see page 112)

Saute onion in a non-stick frypan. Add chicken stock and juice. Mix cornflour with a little water, blend into onion and stock. Stir and cook until smooth. Add tarragon, cook a further 5 minutes. Stir in sour cream just before serving. Pour sauce over each fish fillet and serve with salad. Serves 4.

Fish Parcels with Cashews and Ginger

4 white fish fillets
½ cup roasted unsalted cashews, chopped
1 carrot
1 small zucchini
½ small red pepper
½ small green pepper
2 teas fresh ginger, grated
½ cup fresh breadcrumbs

Sauce
1 cup pineapple juice
1 teas tamari

Combine cashews, vegetables, ginger and breadcrumbs. Cover each piece of fish with a portion of vegetable mixture, fold fish over and secure with a tooth pick. Mix pineapple juice with tamari and pour over fish parcels. Bake in moderate oven for 15 minutes or until fish is tender. Serve with salad. Serves 4.

Golden Prawn Fritters with Lemon Wine Sauce

½ cup self-raising flour
2 egg whites
1 cup skim milk
500 g (1 lb) cooked prawns
1 cup cooked rice
3 shallots, chopped
1 tabs mint, chopped
1 tabs lemon juice

Sift flour, stir in lightly beaten egg whites and milk, then mix in remaining ingredients. Form into balls. Heat a non-stick pan and place heaped tablespoons of mixture into pan. Cook fritters until golden brown, serve with lemon wine sauce (see next page) and salad.

Lemon Wine Sauce

1 egg white
¼ cup lemon juice
½ cup stock
½ cup white wine
2 teas cornflour
2 tabs coriander

Beat egg white until soft peaks form. Gradually add lemon juice. Heat stock and wine in a saucepan, stir in blended cornflour, stir over heat until sauce thickens. Cool, add egg mixture and coriander. Serve with prawn fritters.

Chinese Fish Kebabs

500 g (1 lb) white fish (gem or other thick fish)

Honey Marinade
1 clove garlic, crushed
2 tabs honey
1 tabs coriander, chopped
2 teas fresh ginger, grated
½ cup lemon juice

Combine marinade ingredients in a bowl. Cut fish fillets into large chunks, toss in marinade, refrigerate overnight. Thread fish onto skewers. Barbecue or grill, serve with marinade.

Quick Herb Damper

1 cup self-raising flour
1 onion, chopped
3/4 cup milk
1 cup grated low-fat cheese
2 egg whites
2 tabs chopped herbs

Combine all ingredients and knead on a floured board. Shape into damper shape, place on a greased tray and cook for 30 minutes at 220°C (425°F). Mixture can be made into herb muffins or bread.

Recipe Index